MOMMY, ME,

AND VITAMIN D

(SOMEONE IS COUNTING ON YOU)

By Eugene L Heyden, RN

Impact Health Publishing

Spokane, WA, USA

Impact Health Publishing
Spokane, WA USA

ISBN: 978-0-9828276-3-5

Printed in the United States of America

~For Mom ~

~Contents~

~Preface~

Vitamin D deficiency during pregnancy is the origin of a host of future perils for the child. Some of this damage done by maternal vitamin D deficiency becomes evident after many years. Therefore, prevention of vitamin D deficiency among pregnant women is essential. The current recommended supplementation amount of vitamin D is not sufficient during pregnancy. ~**Kaushal and Magon, 2013**

Vitamin D deficiency and its consequences are extremely subtle, but have <u>enormous</u> implications for human health and disease. It is for this reason that vitamin D deficiency continues to go unrecognized by a majority of health professionals. ~**Holick, 2003, emphasis added**

I n this book we will take a good hard look at the damage done to our children by a simple little thing. Vitamin D deficiency is a simple little thing, but with very serious consequences. It is a preventable cause of so much tragedy and so much heartache. If you are in the business of creating the next generation and have an interest in doing it right, this book is for you. Do not put it down.

Unarguably, the most important job on earth is to provide our children with the best possible start in life, one child at a time. This, of course, is best accomplished before the child is born, perhaps even before the child is conceived. The best start in life is typically a healthy mom living a healthy lifestyle, followed by a well-ordered fetal development with all needs supplied. Remarkably, vitamin D deficiency in "Mom" can screw all this up, and sometimes in a big way. This is the story I will tell. I will also share with you how vitamin D deficiency can harm our children during the various stages of life after birth.

I am still surprised it has taken so long for a book of this nature to come into being. And I can't believe I am the one who has the privilege of writing such a valuable book . . . just for you. As you continue reading, you will see how important vitamin D is to the beginnings and to the life of your child, and you will know exactly what to do. That being said, I am not merely concerned with the health of your child, I am also concerned about your wellbeing.

Unfortunately, this mommy business is risky business. Not only are there unfavorable outcomes related to improper fetal development that the child will bear, perhaps for a lifetime, vitamin D deficiency can also be a threat to you, and in several ways. Harmful, even life-threatening events can occur during pregnancy due to this. In the setting of vitamin D deficiency, your personal risk of several medical conditions greatly increases. We will explore these issues here.

Now, about this book: It will be different. I'll see to that! Although I will give you a sense of what the science is telling us, I will spare you and not go too in-depth, but you will need your thinking cap on! And you will need to be willing to learn a few new things in your quest to provide the best start in life for the one who is counting on you. Here I will expose you to what the physicians and scientists are saying about mommies, babies, and vitamin D. Don't worry, none of this will be hard. And to be extra nice, I will use a little humor to help us out. Books on disease, unfavorable outcomes, and loss of life are not typically enjoyable to read (or write), but we can take the edge off by having a little fun as we travel together through the pages of this book. Let's get started.

~Eugene L. Heyden, RN

Introduction

Calling vitamin D a "vitamin" is something of a misnomer. Although the name is still used for historical reasons, vitamin D is more properly classified as a secosteroid because it consists of a cholesterol backbone and exerts steroid-like effects throughout the body, directly affecting the expression of over 1000 genes through the nuclear vitamin D receptor.
~Cekic et al., 2011

The high prevalence of vitamin D insufficiency during pregnancy is increasingly recognized, amid growing evidence that the intrauterine environment can have both immediate and long-lasting effects on health of the offspring. **~Ponsonby et al., 2010**

Vitamin D intake is <u>essential</u> for maternal health and prevention of adverse outcomes. **~Shin et al., 2010, emphasis added**

So what is vitamin D? And why is it important to the mother-to-be? Sounds quite complicated, but the answer to both questions is rather simple. Vitamin D is a hormone, a hormone necessary for proper development, for proper maintenance and function, and for defense. In essence, it is a hormone necessary for a multitude of favorable genetic events to take place, as needed, and right on schedule. The use of the word vitamin is only appropriate when alluding to the fact that we can obtain this necessary "ingredient" from diet or from supplementation. But when all is said and done, vitamin D is still a hormone, pure and simple. And with respect to the fetus, vitamin D is one very important developmental hormone. It should probably be in adequate supply. Now with that out of the way . . .

This hormone we call a vitamin is produced for us by the largest organ we have, the skin. But more is needed than just skin. Skin needs input. It needs exposure to a certain wavelength of sunlight called UVB radiation in order to create this hormone . . . from cholesterol! Yes, cholesterol! We typically hear the word cholesterol spoken of in a negative light, but cholesterol is *essential* for the creation of several hormones, like estrogen, progesterone, and testosterone. And we all know how important hormones are! Hormones actually "drive" us into this baby-making business. We call it love because that is what it is, but behind the love is the interplay of hormones that create all the magic. And babies are often the result.

We will assume, for the sake of our discussion, that hormones have lead you do certain things, nice things. I won't need to go into all the details here—actually I would like to and others may find it quite fascinating, but time will not allow. You have missed a period or two, giving you a clue that something is up. And soon, very soon, you know for certain that motherhood awaits. How exciting! And, of course, congratulations are in order. But something else is in order. You will need to continually supply the one developing inside all the ingredients it will take to grow and to develop properly. Vitamin D is one of the ingredients that will be needed at each and every step along the way, and in ever increasing amounts. Few emphasize the importance of this, but I will. Vitamin D is more important to fetal development than you can imagine. You will have to make it or you will need to take it.

Vitamin D deficiency (sometimes called vitamin D insufficiency) during pregnancy can lead to a wide variety of disorders, including the loss of fetal life, even the loss of the life of the mother-to-be. So this *is* serious business. But even if the worst does not happen, there are various shades of evil that can occur should the supply of this "hormone" be inadequate to meet the needs of the one who somehow found his or her way inside. Please pay close attention to the story I tell. Someone is counting on you.

Vitamin D insufficiency has been associated with a number of adverse pregnancy outcomes, and has been recognized as a public health concern. (Bener et al., 2013)

In the last 3 years, an increasing amount of research suggests that some of the **damage** done by vitamin D deficiency is done in-utero while the fetus is developing. <u>Much of that damage is permanent</u>, that is, it cannot be fully reversed by taking vitamin D after birth. (Kaushal and Magon, 2013)

Now I think I have your attention.

Behold the gray box!

I love these gray boxes! I use them in all my books. Each gray box I add to the end of a chapter gives me an additional opportunity to discuss with you other things that I feel will contribute significantly to the subject at hand. The gray box will become particularly useful should one want to study a particular subject in depth. And since you need to pay close attention to more than just vitamin D, I will pack the gray box with good things to know. Please pay close attention to the gray box placed at the end of each chapter. I am serious! Did I mention someone is counting on you?

You're going to need this!

There are just a few of concepts and terms to be aware of before we continue. When vitamin D is made from sun exposure, it will eventually be modified to become a molecule called **25(OH)D3**. In the bloodstream, 25(OH)D3 is the circulating form of vitamin D, the molecule that is measured by a blood test with a similar name. This circulating, storage form of vitamin D is converted at the cell level into the "active" form of vitamin D, called **1,25(OH)D2**. If you are taking vitamin D supplements, you have two choices, **D2** or **D3**. D2 is of plant origin. D3 is of animal origin. See how easy this is? Oh! The medical term of a low vitamin D status is **hypovitaminosis D**. Sounds dreadful. It is. You will run across this term a time or two in this presentation. Now you know what it means.

Also, be aware that there is controversy in the medical literature as well as in clinical practice regarding the amount of vitamin D that is actually needed to maintain the health of mice, of humans, of human fetuses, of babies, of just about everyone, including tadpoles of all ages. So expect to find differences in recommendations. Warning: Some who practice medicine are of the belief that we only need a little vitamin D, just about the amount it takes to keep the bones out of trouble plus a little more. However, the research is strongly suggesting that much more than that is needed to maintain overall health and to promote favorable maternal outcomes. This is where I stand. I will present the evidence for this in the pages of this book.

Chapter 1
Before you know it

This . . . hormone also regulates the expression of a large number of genes in reproductive tissues implicating a role for vitamin D in female reproduction.   **~Grundmann and von Versen-Höynk, 2011**

Because of its steroid structure and function, vitamin D plays an important role in priming cells for other hormones to do their action.
~Kaushal and Magon, 2013

Vitamin D deficiency during pregnancy is of epidemic proportions, present in ~20%–85% of women, depending on country of residence and other factors.   **~Shin et al., 2010**

Pregnancy loss is one of the most common obstetric complications, affecting over 30% of conceptions. Most of these occur early in gestation, are due to problems with implantation and may not be clinically apparent.
~Silver, 2007

There is evidence that vitamin D regulates key target genes associated with implantation, trophoblast [recently fertilized egg] invasion and implantation tolerance.   **~Grundmann and von Versen-Höynk, 2011**

So much happens in the life of the fetus before mom has an inkling that she has become host to a new little creature, actually an alien, one who has never been on this earth before now. Well, this is not exactly true. True, it is a little alien, but it was already here, hidden in your genes and in the genes of the other person who somehow became involved. And, of course, hidden in the genes of your parents and of his parents, and of their parents, and of their parents, and so on. The combinations are endless, and a new and unique individual will soon arrive on planet earth in the form of a baby.

Did you know that vitamin D made this all possible? Of course you didn't—you are very busy, occupied with the frivolous things of life. But the truth is, vitamin D is involved not only in the creation of sperm of superior quality, and involved in helping them swim swiftly toward their objective (Lerchbaum and Obermayer-Pietsch, 2012), it is also involved in allowing the fertilized cell to begin the task of developing an interface between it and you (Gundmann and von Versne-Höynic, 2011). This alien will need stuff, so of course a placenta and an umbilical cord will be most necessary—an alien hasta eat, you know! And **you** are on the menu. Some little alien is counting on you.

And being an alien, this new little creature is "foreign" to you. Foreign cells and tissues are generally met with an overwhelming immune reaction, one that recognizes them as undesirable and targets them for destruction. But not now. Your immune system will be "told" not to react, and the alien inside will be allowed to exist and to thrive. This is, in part, under direction of vitamin D, and when supplies are low (think very low) your pregnancy may end at its very beginning, the result of an immune system not all that into alien possession (Shin et al., 2010; Grayson and Hewison, 2011). And another future person is lost forever, destroyed by an immune system that should have been appropriately restrained. But we are getting a little ahead in our story. Rejection is not an issue at this point in time. It is implantation that I am a little worried about (more in a few moments). There are a few crucial events that need to occur or there will be no little alien.

Fertilization of the egg, more formally called the ovum, takes place in the fallopian tube, a passageway leading from ovary to uterus. It is a 3-day journey from fallopian tube to uterus (Lyons et al., 2006). This journey is an assisted journey, assisted by a lining of oscillating hair-like structures that reside on the inner surface of the fallopian tube and gently move the now rapidly dividing egg (blastocyst) forward, in the direction of the uterus (Lyons et al., 2006). Muscular contractions of the fallopian tube also play an important role in moving the fertilized egg toward its goal (Lyons et al., 2006). Apparently, vitamin D plays a role in this journey, but even in those who are deficient, this seems to still go as planned—there must be enough vitamin D around somewhere to pull this off. Although things are headed in the right direction, the pregnancy has not yet begun. Implantation is next on the agenda. Boy I hope this goes well!

Implantation (permanent attachment to the inner lining of the uterus) is a complex series of events involving hormonal signaling between the fertilized egg and the anticipating uterus. And the vitamin D hormone is crucially involved (Shin et al., 2010; Grayson and Hewison, 2011; Gundmann and von Versne-Höynic, 2011). Women with low vitamin D levels have lower rates of implantation success (think infertility) (Shin et al., 2010; Grayson and Hewison, 2011). Even those who undergo what is called artificial or *in vitro* fertilization may fail to become pregnant if vitamin D levels are low (Grayson and Hewison, 2011; Lerchbaum and Obermayer-Pietsch, 2012). However, we do know that pregnancy can occur even in the vitamin D deficient woman, but this is a set-up for compromised fetal development should correction not occur.

Once implantation transpires, vitamin D will be needed in ever-increasing amounts for normal development to take place and for the fulfillment of other important needs that arise during gestation (Dror and Allen, 2010).

So before you know it, a pregnancy has begun. ***Your pregnancy!*** And the outcome of this pregnancy is not at all certain. There are many dangers ahead. One danger is a mother who is ill-informed or inattentive to the needs of the one who is developing deep inside, and developing at an *incredible* rate. You are going to get bigger and just might explode.

Miracle on board

The making of a baby is simply amazing—yes the fun part, but also the developmental part. You are on one *incredible* journey! If you would like to watch a great little video on fetal development, there are many on YouTube to choose from. Start with this one:

—Fetal Development
www.youtube.com/watch?v=AoisqOGQIVE

Diet during pregnancy

When it comes to diet during pregnancy, there is a more to consider than eating wholesome foods and avoiding foods that are tasty but not very nutritious. I'm still trying to figure out how to force you to watch the following video. **You really need to watch this one!** It is produced by the good folks at Parents Magazine, so you know it is exceptional. Search for:

—Healthy Pregnancy Diet
http://www.youtube.com/watch?v=i7ikrxvC1q0

So important!

You have probably already heard of folic acid and its importance during pregnancy. Its use can help reduce a handful of serious birth defects known collectively as neural tube defects. Even though this type of birth defect is not caused by a folate deficiency, per se, boosting ones folate level with folic acid helps influence certain metabolic pathways involved in normal fetal development (Chaudhuri, 2005). (However, a low folate intake, in and of itself, could also lead to neural tube defects.) This is why taking a prenatal vitamin, <u>even before pregnancy</u>, is so important. It will include folic acid and well as other nutrients that will help provide the best start in life, a start that does not include a serious birth defect.

With all the attention given to folic acid in preventing neural tube defects, you might not be aware that a deficiency in a certain vitamin, vitamin B12, is also involved. According to *WebMD*, *"Women with B12 deficiency in early pregnancy were up to five times more likely to have a child with a neural tube defect, such as spina bifida, compared to women with high levels of B12."* (*WebMD*, 2009) So it makes sense to choose a prenatal vitamin that includes B12. It also makes sense to screen women for B12 deficiency, aggressively identifying those who may be at high risk, and performing laboratory testing at any hint of a possible deficiency. For example, those who practice vegetarianism or who are vegan would be at high risk of developing B12 deficiency (Van Sande et al., 2013). Perhaps surprisingly, the absence of the symptoms of B12 deficiency does not assure that a problem does not exist. Diets high in folic acid and folic acid supplementation may mask the symptoms of B12 deficiency, allowing it to remain unidentified unless testing is performed (Selhub et al., 2009; Običan et al., 2010). You are also at an elevated risk for B12 deficiency if you have tummy troubles— have Crohn's disease or celiac disease, have had gastrointestinal surgery (including gastric bypass), or are taking long-term certain medications that reduce stomach acid—so testing seems to be in order under these circumstances (WebMD, 2012; Langan and Zawistoski, 2011). One study found vitamin B12 deficiency in as many as 1 in 20 pregnant women at the earliest stages of pregnancy, a time when neural tube defects occur (Thompson et al., 2009). We're not talkin' rare! This B12 business really is important. You are going to want to discuss this issue with your physician. Tie a string around your finger if that's what it takes.

Vitamin B12 status during pregnancy is critical since maternal B12 deficiency can affect the pregnancy outcome for both mother and the offspring. For women who want to get pregnant, a vitamin B12 deficiency means an increased risk of developing preeclampsia, intra-uterine growthretardation, preterm labor. (Van Sande et al., 2013)

Be ever so careful!

Certain medications can lead to neural tube defects, and do so by **reducing folate levels** (phenytoin, carbamazepine, primidone and phenobarbital) or by **interfering with folate metabolism** (valproic acid). These are drugs that are primarily used to treat epilepsy, and to a lesser extent used for chronic pain and mood disorders (see Hulisz, 2013). Other drugs that may cause neural tube defects include aminopterin, methotrexate, sulfasalazine, triamterene, and trimethoprim (Hernánadez-Díaz et al., 2001). Any of the above-named drugs, if used during the first or second month after the last menstrual period, "*more than doubled*" the risk of neural tube defects (Hernánadez-Díaz et al., 2001). Take a look at the generic name of each drug you are taking. If it matches the name of any of the drugs mentioned above, contact your physician as soon as possible, even if you are not pregnant . . . yet. Nice happens! Neural tube defects occur soon after conception, about two weeks after the first missed period, so be proactive (Hall, 2000). And one more thing.

Surprisingly, smoking, including passive smoking, can also lead to neural tube defects (Suarez et al., 2007). This is one of the many good reasons why quitting smoking during the child-bearing years is so important.   (Someone is counting on you not to be a smoker.)

Have I got an app for you!

Now, on the lighter side—and we're talkin' fun! I have this great little app installed on my iPad. It includes images covering the various stages of fetal development, week by week, plus so much more. It is produced by Pampers—you're going to be singing the praises of this company several times a day! The app is called **_Hello Baby_**.   It is available from iTunes and Google Play (for android devices). It is a free app, fun, and, may I add, very worthwhile.

Chapter 2
Everything should be just fine

The present study demonstrated a greater risk of maternal complications in pregnant women with vitamin D deficiency compared with those with normal vitamin D levels. **~Bener et al., 2013**

The fetus relies <u>entirely</u> on the vitamin D stores of the mother, so if the mother is deficient, so is the fetus. **~Bodnar et al., 2007a, emphasis added**

The vitamin D-deficiency epidemic during pregnancy is caused by a lack of adequate sunlight exposure needed to synthesize vitamin D in the skin, coupled with overall intakes that are too low to meet the increased demands of pregnancy. **~Berner et al., 2013**

Well, the alien has landed, and has successfully created a lifeline connecting itself to its host—it needs stuff! This little creature will do everything else, all by itself—growth, development, and possibly sprouting an impressive head of hair—as long as it *extracts* what it needs from Mom. But this little guy or gal (yes, the gender has already been determined) has landed on a hostile planet. There are other aliens in the neighborhood that, for some reason, want to end its life. A battle is now occurring—one that you unknowingly wage—a battle against the enemies of the little alien whom you will love to pieces and give a cute little name. The battle is constant, it is fierce, and it is directed against bacteria that are evil.

Although the uterus is regarded as a sterile environment, this may not always be the case. It is only a "sterile" environment due to the fierce actions of the mother's immune system (Fahey et al., 2006). Vitamin D orchestrates this host defense, somehow knowing there is someone very valuable inside that it needs to protect. Surprisingly, Mom is relying on beneficial bacteria living in her vagina to out-compete harmful bacteria for space and nutrients and in this manner block their advance (Gundmann and von Versne-Höynic, 2011; Dover et al., 2008). But for the bacteria that dare advance toward the one developing inside, there awaits a nasty little surprise. It is a molecule called cathelicidin. Bacteria tremble in fear when it is near. It is out to kill them.

Cathelicidin is a natural antibiotic that kills on contact and defends against infection along the entire reproductive tract (Shin et al., 2010). In addition to the cells that line this tract, there is an army of immune cells that reside just below the surface, ready to "eat" and destroy any bacteria that come their way. Vitamin D is necessary for cathelicidin production, and stimulates certain immune cells to kill and to keep on killing (Shin et al., 2010; Grayson and Hewison, 2011). A lot of killing is involved in making a baby, but you never know any of this is occurring. It is a silent war, but it is war, nevertheless. When vitamin D supplies are low, the mothers' ability to wage this war and protect her unborn child is compromised. Cathelicidin production, and release, is reduced, and many, many innocent little ones are lost due to this unfortunate turn of events. Surprisingly, the ball of cells that arises from and surrounds the rapidly dividing fertilized egg—and travels to the uterus for implantation (and from which the embryo arises)—uses cathelicidin as needed in its personal battle against bacteria. These amazing cells can actually eat a bacterium and destroy it within, all by the stimulatory and antibacterial actions of this natural antibiotic (Liu et al., 2009; Choy and Manyonda, 1998). Your baby, even before it becomes an embryo, is a killer. It desperately wants to survive on this hostile planet. It will do anything! And it is hoping vitamin D will be in adequate supply.

Well, we can breathe a sigh of relief knowing that vitamin D supplies seem to be adequate for the moment. The little alien is now firmly attached to its host. It is growing at an *impressive* rate and so are the structures that will support its needs for the next 9 months. The hormone called vitamin D helps orchestrate the growth and development of the placenta and other structures that transport "stuff." Vitamin D deficiency compromises this interface between alien and host. And if this interface is compromised enough, the pregnancy will be lost. We call this a miscarriage.

A miscarriage can occur for a variety of reasons. It actually occurs quite frequently (ending 15–20% of all pregnancies in the US) and is *most* unfortunate. But it is less unfortunate than the alternative . . . sometimes. A miscarriage, although tragic, is sometimes nature's way of saying "Sorry, but the one developing inside is too compromised to survive should the pregnancy continue." Regardless of the cause, this is a time of great sadness. Someone is lost forever.

Well, according to our story, vitamin D has so far been adequate, and things seem to be going quite well for the little alien, at least for the moment. Mom will still be "consuming" or creating vitamin D to meet her needs, but she will also be supplying the vitamin D needs of someone else, someone who needs "stuff." And the demands for vitamin D start to climb. But the typical "Mom" is already vitamin D deficient, so expect a lot of problems to occur in the pregnant population. One such problem is called preeclampsia. There are other problems common in those who are deficient in vitamin D. Let's take a look at the major ones, one by one.

Preeclampsia

Preeclampsia, as identified by new onset hypertension [high blood pressure] and proteinuria [protein spilling into the urine] during pregnancy, is a serious disorder affecting 5–8% of pregnancies, and is alleviated only by delivery of the placenta. **~Shin et al., 2010**

In a recent study, the odds of severe preeclampsia decreased by 38% for every 10 nmol/L increase in 25(OH)D.

Interestingly, the odds of developing preeclampsia were reduced by 51% in women who received high dose (2,000 IU/day) vitamin D supplement during their first year of life. **~Christensen et al., 2012**

Women with vitamin D deficiency (<20 ng/ml) were more likely to have low levels of placental growth factor, which is associated with an increased risk of preeclapsia. **~Fanos et al., 2013**

Preeclampsia is serious business, risky business. It apparently affects up to 10% of all pregnancies (Backes et al., 2011; Liu et al., 2011). *"Recent evidence suggests that preeclampsia accounts for approximately 15.9% of all maternal deaths in the United States and is a major cause of perinatal morbidity and death."* (Backes et al., 2011) A recent study found that *"patients with 25(OH)D levels 15 ng/mL [quite low, but common] had a* **5-fold increase** *in the risk of preeclampsia, despite receiving prenatal vitamins."* (Mulligan et al., 2010, emphasis added) It certainly seems that vitamin D deficiency is a major risk factor for preeclampsia. So what exactly is preeclampsia and why should it be avoided?

"Preeclampsia is a collection of symptoms during pregnancy that are linked to maternal hypertension [high blood pressure]." (Grayson and Hewison, 2011) It is a serious turn of events for both mother and developing fetus, generally occurring after 20 weeks of gestation. And it *is* serious. Occasionally, a mother will die. Many times a pregnancy is lost. Evidence suggests *"a strong link between vitamin D insufficiency and preeclampsia."* (Grayson and Hewison, 2011) The tipoff is a rise in "Mom's" usual blood pressure.

The effect of preeclampsia on the mother ranges from no symptoms at all, to severe, debilitating symptoms. And the fetus is left wondering if it will even survive. Science is still trying to figure things out, with speculation that preeclampsia is related to abnormalities of the placenta, is related to immune system dysfunction, is involved in the regulation of blood pressure, and so on. (Pérez-López, 2007) Not surprisingly, vitamin D is involved in the proper growth of the placenta, proper immune system function, the regulation of blood pressure, and so on. Preeclampsia can be a challenge for the physician, and what should be a normal pregnancy has now been transformed into a high-risk pregnancy. Its occurrence is a sign that blood flow to the fetus is compromised and bad things could happen (Backes et al., 2011). **The infant born of a preeclamptic mother may be born too early, and is 5 times more likely to die** (Lain and Roberts, 2002). And, yes, vitamin D deficiency can be at least somewhat responsible, at least sometimes, perhaps many times (Pérez-López, 2007; Bodnar et al., 2007a).

By now, I'm guessing you don't want anything to do with preeclampsia. Good call! If things get out of control, a more serious, life-threating disorder called eclampsia will follow. I won't go into all the details here, but you probably don't want anything to do with this thing either. Eclampsia is very, <u>very</u> serious business. It is basically an intensification of the symptoms of preeclampsia, and its adverse effects, with a seizure in "Mom" signaling that things have now escalated to a very dangerous level.

> This is a life-threatening situation for both you and your baby. During a seizure, you and your baby are at risk of being deprived of oxygen. In addition, the high blood pressure may cause the placenta to separate from the wall of the uterus, called placental abruption. This can cause severe bleeding and even death of the fetus and possibly the mother. (*Web*MD, 2013a)

Thank goodness eclampsia is rare (1 in every 2,000 to 3,448 pregnancies in Western countries according to the online journal MD CONSULT). It is rare thanks to the great care directed at managing preeclampsia. But less of this great care would be needed if we as a society, physicians and mothers included, were to pay more attention to vitamin D. Recall, preeclampsia is **5-fold** more prevalent in those who are vitamin D deficient (Mulligan et al., 2010). Therefore, since preeclampsia is 5 times more prevalent in mothers who are low in vitamin D, it follows that eclampsia, which stems from preeclampsia, is at least 5 times more likely to occur in those who are vitamin D deficient. (I did the math all by myself.)

Of course, the more "on her toes" the mother is, the better prenatal care she can receive. Promptly report any of the following: Rapid weight gain (2-5 pounds in a single week) swelling of the face or arms, headaches, any visual disturbance, dizziness of faintness, ringing in the ears, abdominal pain, the onset of nausea or vomiting, blood in urine or emesis, periods of confusion, or a seizure. (see *WebMD*, 2013b) Let's move on, I've had it with preeclampsia.

Well, I guess I do have a little more to say about preeclampsia after all. Surprisingly, if a woman received 2,000 IU/day of vitamin D in her first year of life, her risk of contracting preeclampsia, <u>when she herself becomes pregnant</u>, is reduced by half! (Huh and Gordon, 2008; Christesen et al., 2012) Apparently, there are long-lasting benefits of vitamin D supplementation during infancy. It paves the way for babies to become the mommies of healthy babies later in life.

One more thing. I didn't dwell nearly enough on the adverse consequences of preeclampsia for the offspring. I'm just sure of it! At the very least, I should at least bring this to your attention:

> Preeclampsia can prevent the placenta from receiving enough blood, which can cause your baby to be born very small. It is also one of the leading causes of premature births, and the complications that can follow, including **learning disabilities, epilepsy, cerebral palsy, hearing and vision problems**. (*WebMD*, 2012, emphasis added)

Another one more thing:

Epidemiological studies show that infants exposed to preeclampsia during gestation are associated with an increased risk of diabetes and cardiovascular morbidity in adulthood. These studies underscore the concept that the physiologically immature fetus is highly susceptible to disruptions *in utero* blood flow and that insults from preeclampsia exposure accrued during critical periods of fetal development may predispose an individual to an increased risk of disease beyond the immediate postnatal period. (Backes et al., 2011)

I think it best to avoid preeclampsia. Vitamin D sufficiency has been shown to help, not in all studies but in enough studies to grab my attention and the attention of many others.

Bacterial vaginosis

In recent studies we have shown that vitamin D is a potent stimulator of innate antimicrobial responses to infection in human placental cells, whilst simultaneously inhibiting inflammation and risk of preterm birth.
~Grayson and Hewiston, 2011

Vitamin D may influence the course of infectious diseases during pregnancy. Low 25(OH)D levels are correlated with increased bacterial vaginosis in the first trimester. Bacterial vaginosis is more prevalent in black women, who typically have lower serum 25(OH)D concentrations and have a six-fold higher chance of vitamin D deficiency, compared with white women. **~Kaushal and Magon, 2013**

This sounds about as bad as it probably is. Somehow, bacteria that are evil have gained a foot-hold and are threatening the pregnancy, both the mother and the alien inside. We've talked of this before, but it bears repeating (because it harms and kills babies and makes people very sad).

Vitamin D deficiency has been strongly implicated in this complication of pregnancy. This should come as no surprise, in as much as vitamin D is intimately involved in our defense against bacteria. Remember cathelicidin, the killer molecule bacteria tremble in fear of? This molecule is but one of the many defenses that we could justifiably call *"D-pendent"* on adequate availability of vitamin D. Vitamin D, in effect, turns the placenta into an immunological weapon, a killing machine, one driven to protect the fetus from death by infection (Ben-Hur et al., 2001; Dunlop et al., 2011). Bacteria that threaten the pregnancy have a more difficult time doing so when supplies of vitamin D are plentiful. They get to die! Vitamin D deficiency only invites trouble. The invitation goes out to hoards of harmful bacteria that can't wait to conquer and live to destroy. And they don't mind killing the innocent. They are bad. Vitamin D has the power to protect and to save (by killing), but it will need to be in adequate supply or problems could arise.

One important thing to keep in mind: bacterial vaginosis can lead to infections of fluids and structures that are in immediate contact with the fetus (Yoon et al., 2003). This is a big threat to the little alien (aka your future little bundle of joy). It can lead to birth defects, including the birth defect of being born too early (Yoon et al., 2003.) *"Approximately 25–40% of all preterm births are thought to be associated with intrauterine infection."* (Thorne-Lyman and Fawzi, 2012) Prematurity can make for a rough start in life. It can also take a life.

Gestational diabetes mellitus (GDM)

Vitamin D deficiency during early pregnancy significantly increases the risk for gestational diabetes in later pregnancy.   ~**Kaushal and Magon, 2013**

Gestational diabetes is a result of pregnancy-induced insulin resistance and impaired compensating insulin secretion. Vitamin D improves insulin sensitivity by enhancing insulin responsiveness to glucose transport.
~Berner et al., 2013

Gestational diabetes mellitus (GDM) is clearly related to vitamin D deficiency—not always, but a good share of the time. It affects 14% of all pregnancies in the United States and can increase the risk of a surgical delivery and of type 2 diabetes later in "Mom" later on (Burris et al., 2012). The baby is also adversely affected by GDM. *"GDM leads to excess fetal insulin production; insulin acts as a growth factor causing increased fetal size and relative amount of fat mass."* (Josefson et al., 2013) Baby fat is, of course, cute—but when created in excess, and created by the gestational diabetes of "Mom," it may set the stage for a chubby little life to continue being a chubby little life . . . forever! (Gillman et al., 2003; Walsh et al., 2012) Besides a heavier little bundle of joy, which can cause birth trauma to both mother and newborn, GDM can lead to respiratory distress, jaundice, and low blood sugar in the new baby (Burris et al., 2012).

The risk of GDM is **2.7 times greater** if Mom's 25OHD level is <20 ng/mL, according to one study (Gundmann and von Versne-Höynic, 2011). Vitamin D is involved in GDM due to its influence on insulin secretion and its positive influence on the responsiveness to insulin by the insulin receptor (Zhang et al., 2010; Zuhr et al., 2013). Certainly, there are other factors involved, but clearly less of this GDM business would occur if our population were sufficient in vitamin D.

A recent study suggests that <u>only</u> those severely deficient in vitamin D during pregnancy have an increased risk of GDM (Zuhur et al., 2013). But don't relax. There are plenty of severely vitamin deficient people around. You could be one of them. Have you been tested? People often come up to me reporting their surprise to having just found out that their vitamin D level was extremely low and they are among the walking dead. It takes a blood test to make sure you are truly vitamin D sufficient. If you are deficient, it will show you just how deficient you are. Ask for one today. Insist!

Vitamin D is important to maternal health, fetal development, and postnatal life. Current prenatal care does not include the monitoring of vitamin D levels, which is an unfortunate oversight because deficiency is easily treated. (Mulligan et al., 2010)

Impaired fetal growth and prematurity

Fetal growth is a useful marker of fetal well-being. Pregnancies complicated by intrauterine growth restriction, defined as a pathological process of reduced fetal growth, have been associated with an increase in perinatal mortality. **~Backes et al., 2011**

Sometimes a baby is born too small, its growth impaired by many factors including vitamin D deficiency in Mom, and Mom may find herself in the scrawny little baby business (Pérez-López, 2007). Even this is risky business! We should consider low birth weight as a birth defect. It represents a level of immaturity that can challenge the little one after birth, and sometimes for quite some time.

A premature birth makes for an ill-prepared start in life. Even the so called *late-preterm* infant can get into a lot of trouble (Backes et al., 2011). All of the major medical conditions discussed thus far— preeclampsia, gestational diabetes, bacterial vaginosis—can lead to a birth that occurs ahead of schedule. And being born just a little early is not without risk.

Even the *late-term* or *near-term* infant, previously thought to be as *"good as ready,"* is <u>not</u> ready. *"Evidence suggests than late-preterm infants have a **nine times** greater incidence of respiratory distress syndrome that term infants."* (Backes et al., 2011, emphasis added) A *late-preterm* birth is one that occurs between 34 to 36 weeks gestation (4 to 6 weeks too early). But what about a birth that occurs before this period of time? Well, the risks only increase, and a lot of excellent (and expensive) medical care will be required. And it's not just respiratory difficulties that occur in greater frequency due to prematurity; premature babies are at greater risk of infections, jaundice, anemia, and visual impairment, to name a few (source: March of Dimes). And, as bad as all of this is, this is just the little stuff. Try living the life of the individual afflicted with cerebral palsy . . . for a lifetime! Prematurity, occurring for a variety of reasons, increases the risk of this *dreadful* condition. Surprisingly, *"Cerebral palsy, with a prevalence of 2 to 2.5 per 1,000 live births, is the most common severe physical disability affecting children."* (Hutton and Pharoah, 2006) And preeclampsia, leading to prematurity, is a major risk factor for cerebral palsy. We should do our best to prevent it.

> Children exposed to preeclampsia and born small for gestational age had a significantly increased risk of cerebral palsy. (Strand et al., 2013, emphasis added)

> The leading risk factor for cerebral palsy is prematurity. The prevalence of cerebral palsy at age 3 years is 44 per 1000 born at <27 weeks, 21 per 1000 for those born between 28 and 30 weeks, and 0.6 per 1000 for those delivered at term. (Yoon et al., 2003)

Is vitamin D deficiency a risk factor for cerebral palsy? Perhaps so indirectly—via placental insufficiency, impaired defense against infection, or impaired fetal growth—all factors related to vitamin D deficiency and leading to prematurity. If vitamin D sufficiency can reduce the incidence of contributing risk factors for cerebral palsy, it should probably be included as a risk factor in its own right. Which brings us to the next topic of discussion.

Birth defects and vitamin D

Complications that can follow premature birth include learning disabilities, epilepsy, cerebral palsy, and hearing and vision problems. **~WebMD, 2012, paraphrased**

In the last 3 years, an increasing amount of research suggests that some of the damage done by vitamin D deficiency is done in-utero while the fetus is developing. ***Much of that damage is permanent****, that is, it cannot be fully reversed by taking vitamin D after birth.* **~Kaushal and Magon, 2013, emphasis added**

So what could some of this damage be? In addition to contributing to prematurity (which, in turn, increases the risk of cerebral palsy, learning disabilities, epilepsy, and hearing and visual problems) other issues associated with a low vitamin D status in Mom have been reported.

Low maternal vitamin D status may slow neonatal cardiac development and alter brain morphology (structure), with changes in the latter persisting into adulthood. (Ponsonby et al., 2010)

The vitamin D status of a mother-to-be is starting to sound like something very important to pay close attention to. Yet, in our society, we leave vitamin D sufficiency up to chance, hoping Mom will get enough sun (which usually doesn't happen), hoping that Mom will drink enough D-fortified milk or orange juice (which never really occurs), hoping that Mom will take her vitamin-D-deficient prenatal vitamin (which she probably will, although it will make no real difference), and hoping that mom will be totally healthy and will be living a healthy lifestyle (good luck with that!). Later, you will learn just how easy it is to become vitamin D deficient or <u>very</u> vitamin D deficient, and you won't even know it (and likely neither will your physician unless he or she is being watchful and testing for it). Sadly, if vitamin D deficiency is not caught in those who are or may become pregnant, bad things can happen. It can lead to a son or to a daughter who has special needs and special difficulties, some that last for a lifetime. Heard of autism? Heard of schizophrenia? Yes, vitamin D deficiency in Mom can lead to these unfavorable, sometimes devastating outcomes. I will present evidence for this in a later chapter.

Apparently the heart, the lungs, and the brain are developmentally at risk in the offspring should "Mom" be deficient in vitamin D. The extent of the damage is unknown. But we are beginning to take notice.

> Research in cardiology suggests that gestational vitamin D deficiency may be a determinate of preventable infant heart failure, while respiratory research suggests an association between lower respiratory infections in newborns with vitamin D inadequacy likely arising from maternal insufficiency. There is the concern about insufficient vitamin D as a possible factor contributing to the sky rocketing rates of autistic spectrum disorder. (Grant et al., 2010)

The ultimate birth defect, however, may be a life that can no longer be lived or a life that is suddenly swept away. The death of a baby can, of course, occur before birth, and there is great sadness throughout the land. Vitamin D deficiency during pregnancy can be a contributing factor, the research is clear. *"Vitamin D concentrations were significantly lower in women . . . who had an intrauterine fetal death."* (Shand et al., 2010) But imagine the sadness felt when an apparently healthy, normal baby is suddenly lost in the first year or so of life. I, personally, have heard the cry of a mother who had just lost her baby to SIDS (sudden infant death syndrome), and I never want to hear *anything* like it again.

There is compelling evidence that SIDS (aka crib death) <u>may be</u> related to maternal vitamin D deficiency. More investigational work will be needed before we know more fully the role vitamin D plays in SIDS, but, remarkably, one team of investigators found that in babies who suddenly pass away during the first year of life, **<u>87% had evidence of rickets</u>**, a disease primarily caused by severe vitamin D deficiency (Post and Ernst, 2013; Cohen et al., 2013).   In rickets, the bones are soft and misshapen, and generally <u>only</u> occurs when vitamin D availability is very low. This is a major finding!

The sooner we end this chapter the better—it is ripping my heart out. Let's close with this:

> Considering the adverse effects of maternal vitamin D deficiency on offspring such as neonatal hypocalcemia [low calcium level], seizure, impaired development and rickets, the high prevalence of hypovitaminosis D [vitamin D deficiency] during pregnancy is a major health problem, and **vitamin D supplementation during pregnancy is of paramount importance**. (Zuhur et al., 2013, emphasis added)

Yes, I have another baby book

Let me tell you about another book I wrote. It is entitled ***Preventing Birth Defects: Understanding the Iodine/Thyroid Hormone Connection***. Why would I write such a book? It is because you are so unaware that iodine and thyroid hormone insufficiency destroys the lives of so many babies, babies who have the right to be born healthy and free of physical and intellectual defect. Someone needs to warn you of some of this:

> Normal maternal thyroid function during pregnancy is <u>critical</u> for fetal development. **Deficient maternal thyroid hormone levels during pregnancy are associated with impaired neuropsychological development in childhood, premature birth, preeclampsia, and fetal mortality.**
> (Burnam, 2009, emphasis added)

> *All degrees of iodine deficiency . . . affect thyroid function of the mother and the neonate as well as the mental development of the child. (Delange, 2001, emphasis added)*

Iodine deficiency increases neonatal mortality. **We emphasize this statement so that iodine deficiency can take its proper place among disorders that kill children.** (Dunn and Delange, 2001, emphasis added)

Many birth defects, including cleft palate, cerebral palsy, and mental retardation are clearly related to iodine and thyroid hormone insufficiency. You need to know the story. You need to know how vulnerable your baby really is.

Preventing Birth Defects: Understanding the Iodine/Thyroid Hormone Connection is quite a book. My goal is to have it in print this year, 2014. Look for it. Someone is counting on you to not only look for it but also to read it. I will announce its arrival on my website (unless I forget).

Chapter 3
Not up to the task

The vitamin D-deficiency epidemic is caused by a lack of adequate sunlight exposure needed to synthesize vitamin D3 in skin, coupled with overall intakes that are too low to meet the increasing demand of pregnancy. **~Berner et al., 2013**

Vitamin D deficiency during pregnancy is the origin of a host of future perils for the child. **Some of this damage done by maternal vitamin D deficiency becomes evident after many years.** *Therefore, prevention of vitamin D deficiency among pregnant women is essential. The current recommended supplementation amount of vitamin D is not sufficient during pregnancy.* **~Kaushal and Magon, 2013, emphasis added**

As vitamin D status in the mother and fetus is closely correlated, vitamin D deficient mothers will give birth to vitamin D deficient infants. **~Hyppönen, 2011**

I see trouble ahead.

When "Mom" is vitamin D deficient, so is the one who is developing inside, the one who will continue to develop after birth—and vitamin D is a <u>key</u> developmental hormone, one that we <u>cannot</u> do without. Sure, a mother may be able to squeak by (maybe), supplying only minimal amounts of this "hormone" to meet the needs of her baby with no noticeable ill effects, but damage does occur to many babies due to vitamin D deficiency. Pregnancies are lost, and unfavorable outcomes— some unnoticeable but still present—are commonplace when the supply of this hormone is not up to the task. And **the only one that can really do anything about it is the mother herself**. We need this little talk. We can start with your prenatal vitamin.

Prenatal vitamin deficiency

Despite the fact that pregnant women in most countries are encouraged to take a daily prenatal supplementation containing vitamin D, a disturbingly high prevalence of hypovitaminosis D [low vitamin D) has been demonstrated amongst pregnant women in nearly all populations studied.   **~Dror and Allen, 2010**

*Infants who are vitamin D deficient at birth are at the highest risk of impaired bone development that appears to persist even in later childhood. What is most concerning is that **use of prenatal vitamins containing 400 IU/tablet was <u>irrelevant</u>** in affecting vitamin D status: those who took their prescribed prenatal vitamin D did not differ from those who did not. Women taking their prenatal vitamins should be counseled that the amount of vitamin D in their prenatal vitamins will not affect their vitamin D status.*   **~Hamilton et al., 2010, emphasis added**

In the United states, $25(OH)D_3$ concentrations are surprisingly low during pregnancy, despite some supplementation with prenatal vitamins. **~Patrick and Ames, 2014**

If you are expecting great things from the vitamin D content of your prenatal vitamin, you can forget it—**even your prenatal vitamin has a vitamin D deficiency!** The tiny amount of vitamin D added to your prenatal (usually 400 IU/tablet) may help . . . somewhat—and obviously some is better than none—but relying on 400 units per day to correct vitamin D deficiency is an exercise in futility. You *certainly* need a prenatal in order to ensure that you do not become deficient in other nutrients, particularly folic acid, but not to achieve and maintain vitamin D sufficiency. It won't work! (Hollis and Wagner, 2004; Hamilton et al., 2010) Even eating a diet rich in vitamin D-enriched foods, plus a prenatal vitamin, may not be enough (Hamilton et al., 2010). It takes regular sun exposure, and/or generous vitamin D supplementation to achieve a vitamin D level that is sufficient, truly sufficient. And if you are significantly overweight *and* pregnant, more aggressive action will be needed (Bodnar et al., 2007b; Holick, 2004). We will discuss recommendations later. By the way, I can say all of this because the experts are saying all of this.

To be fair, the prescribing physician is likely anticipating that the vitamin D dose in a prenatal will probably be enough "just to make sure," because we have D-fortified milk (are you drinking 40 glasses of milk per day?). And besides, people are making plenty of vitamin D just by going outdoors. The truth is, nobody is that thirsty, and we live in a society that typically limits our exposure to sunlight between the hours of the day when vitamin D can be manufactured. Creating vitamin D from sunlight requires sunlight exposure typically between the hours of 10 AM to 3 PM (Rathi and Rathi, 2011). Clearly, a prenatal vitamin—relied upon by many to insure vitamin D sufficiency in both mother and developing fetus—is not up to the task. Clearly! But you don't have to take my word for it. You can take their word for it:

> Finally, let us discuss a scenario that occurs thousands of times daily in the United States. A pregnant woman visits her obstetrician, who prescribes prenatal vitamins containing 400 IU (10µg) vitamin D. The patient and physician both assume that this supplement will fulfill all the nutritional requirements for the duration of the pregnancy. However, in the case of vitamin D, it will not even come close unless the pregnant woman has adequate sun exposure. The woman, especially if African American, and her developing fetus are at high risk of remaining vitamin D deficient during the entire pregnancy. Even if the physician were to prescribe a vitamin D supplement of 1,000 IU/d (25 µg), the mother would likely remain vitamin D deficient. As scientists and health care providers, we simply cannot accept this any longer. (Hollis and Wagner, 2004)

I don't want you to have to wait for another terrific chapter to come along before you come to the realization that you are going to need a lot more vitamin D (thousands of units per day) than the current recommendation, a recommendation that will almost guarantee that you will remain vitamin D deficient throughout your pregnancy. I want you to be aware of this . . . **NOW!** And, of course, do something about it . . . **NOW!** Consider this:

> In the United States, the current recommendation for vitamin D intake during pregnancy is 200–400 IU/d. However, a previous study has shown that prenatal supplements that contain 400 IU of vitamin D are not adequate to achieve normal vitamin D levels in pregnant women or their infants. Even more concerning, studies of supplementation with 800–1,600 IU vitamin D per day during the last trimester of pregnancy in women with 25(OH)D levels <15 ng/mL showed that vitamin D levels increased from 5.8 ng/mL to a mere 11 ng/mL. Therefore, supplemental vitamin D in doses that exceed 1000 IU per day (2,000–10,000 IU/d) may be required to achieve a normal concentration of circulating vitamin D in severely deficient patients. Studies with 2,000–4,000 IU daily of vitamin D supplementation in nonpregnant women have shown these amounts to be safe and effective at achieving normal vitamin D levels. Studies in pregnant women are underway in the United States that use vitamin D at doses of 2,000 IU and 4,000 IU daily to establish vitamin D recommendations during pregnancy. (Mulligan et al., 2010)

Are you getting the point? Thousands of units of vitamin D, not hundreds, will be necessary to achieve a vitamin D level that will be sufficient to meet your needs and the needs of the alien inside.

Before we move on, I need to point this out: If your vitamin D status is sufficient at the end of summer, you may become deficient mid-winter, and remain deficient until the following spring or summer (unless you supplement in relevant amounts). The reason: You can only generate vitamin D in mainland USA between the months of April and September, with some exceptions (Bodnar et al., 2007c). A satisfactory vitamin D test result, during or at the end of summer, will be no guarantee that your current level of supplementation (0, 400, 600, 1000, even 2,000 IU per day) will keep your vitamin D at a satisfactory level throughout your entire pregnancy. I see trouble ahead.

Prenatal care not up to the task?

Vitamin D is important to maternal health, fetal development, and postnatal life. Current prenatal care does not include the monitoring of vitamin D levels, which is an <u>unfortunate oversight</u> because deficiency is easily treated. **~Mulligan et al., 2010, emphasis added**

Vitamin D deficiency is often clinically unrecognized, however laboratory measurements are easy to perform, and treatment of vitamin D deficiency is inexpensive. **~Grundermann and von Versen-Höynck, 2011**

I hate to be the one to break this to you, but your prenatal care may not be up to the task. I, and many others, take issue with the fact that only casual attention is paid to vitamin D, as seen in the "typical" clinical OB/GYN setting (as if vitamin D sufficiency is optional). And whenever I hear headlines such as *"Pregnant Women Don't Need Vitamin D Screening"* in the lay or medical press, I cringe, and so should you. Clearly, more attention to the vitamin D status of "Mom" is needed, a lot more than asking a question or two regarding risk factors for deficiency, more than prescribing a prenatal vitamin, more than sending the patient on her way without clear instruction on how vitamin D sufficiency is achieved and how it is maintained, and hoping for the best. What is needed is <u>routine</u> laboratory testing—best performed before conception and *certainly* performed during early pregnancy. Mid and late pregnancy are also good times to test. Testing is the <u>only</u> way to determine if one is sufficient or deficient in vitamin D, and to what degree (Holick, 2004). In the next chapter, I will share with you what vitamin D sufficiency is and how it is achieved. Someone is counting on you to read the next chapter. But first, someone is counting on you finish this chapter.

Vitamin D deficiency and its consequences are extremely subtle, but have <u>enormous</u> implications for human health and disease. It is for this reason that vitamin D deficiency continues to go unrecognized by a majority of health professionals. (Holick, 2003, emphasis added)

The above was written over 10 years ago. In the meantime, little has changed.

Imagine **YOU** not up to the task

A two to four times higher risk of caesarian delivery was associated to low maternal vitamin D levels in recent years. Observational studies suggest that vitamin D deficiency would undermine pelvic muscle strength and thus pushing ability at delivery, as well as preventing the initiation of labor, which depends on high serum calcium. **~Fanos et al., 2013, emphasis added**

In most infants, vitamin D stores acquired from the mother [in utero] are depleted by approximately 8 weeks of age.

Recent studies show that maternal vitamin D intake of 4,000 IU daily during lactation in vitamin D-in-sufficient mothers enhances vitamin D levels in breast milk and may be a potential therapeutic intervention to prevent vitamin D deficiency-related complications in both women and their breast-fed infants. **~Mulligan et al., 2010**

Women who are vitamin D deficient are at special risk of not having what it takes to deliver their baby the natural (oh so painful) way. Furthermore, the vitamin D deficient mom may not be up to the task of supplying the hungry new little one with enough "developmental" hormone (vitamin D) to adequately meet his or her needs. Exclusive breast feeding is a risk factor for vitamin D deficiency for your baby, but only if, at the same time, you are and you remain vitamin D deficient (Mirsa et al., 2008; Balasubramanian and Ganesh, 2008). But before you can breast feed, you will first need to give birth. (I figured this out all on my own.) I sure hope you are up to the task.

C-section risk

> Vitamin D deficiency is associated with suboptimal muscle performance and strength, which may lead to dystocia [difficult birth] and poor progress during labor. ~Christesen et al., 2012

I previously warned you that this mommy business is risky business. Your risk of requiring an operation to deliver your baby is significantly increased if you are vitamin D deficient. The operation in question is called a C-section, and it is not the easy way out. It hurts, too. And it is not without some risk to mom, including the risk of infection. Surprisingly, it is also risky business for the baby, but in a subtle, surprising way. And just like that, I have another important story to tell.

Among other things, a vaginal birth is nature's way of transferring normal, beneficial bacteria to the baby during the birthing process (Neu and Rushing, 2011). As the baby swallows fluids obtained from passage through the birth canal, he or she begins the process of populating the bowel with bacteria that are good. The good bacteria will establish colonies that act to prevent bad bacteria from establishing a foothold; and will "teach" the baby's immune system how to recognize bacteria that are good and how to recognize and deal with those that are evil. The composition of the bacterial flora in the newborn bowel becomes abnormal following delivery by C-section, and the new little one begins postnatal life with bacteria acquired from the skin rather than the birth canal (Dominguez-Bello et al., 2010). The skin bacteria are more likely to be evil, or at least not represent the bacterial mix that will offer the greatest benefit to the newborn. This *does* make a difference, and several diseases occur more frequently in those who are delivered surgically compared to those who make it out the intended way (Neu and Rushing, 2011). So, C-section should be avoided, if at all possible. Vitamin D sufficiency can help. By the way, it has been determined that a vitamin D level below 15 ng/ml—low to very low—increases the C-section risk **4-fold** compared to those who are vitamin D sufficient. (Dror and Allen, 2010). This is a very significant finding.

Breast feeding not up to the task?

> *For a lactating mother, it is essential that sustained circulating vitamin D be maintained.*

> *We understand more fully now that this deficiency [hypovitaminosis D associated with breastfeeding] is not caused by something inherently wrong or missing in mother's milk but rather by inadequate maternal dietary vitamin D intake and the resultant low concentrations in the mother's milk.* **~Wagner et al., 2008, emphasis added**

> *Although human milk is the best source of nutrition for term infants, vitamin D content of breast milk is insufficient to meet the recommended intake of vitamin D.* **~Mirsa et al., 2008**

It's hard to beat breast milk—I could use some now! It is chock full of nutrients and does a body good. It is *exactly* what your baby needs (so I'll pass on the offer), but breast milk may not be up to the task of providing enough vitamin D for your baby if you are D-ficient (Misra et al., 2008). The more vitamin D "Mom" makes or takes, the more she will be able to pass on to little Jimmy (or little Suzie or whomever the little alien has turned into).

If "Mom" is not creating relevant amounts of vitamin D from sun exposure (like who has the time for that, with a brand new baby and all?), she *will* need to supplement with vitamin D. No doubt about it. A dose of 400 or 600 units per day from a vitamin tablet will not be enough. A 1,000 IU/day dose may bring you from the deficiency range into the insufficiency range, but it is unlikely to be nearly enough to meet the needs of the one who is nursing (Wagner et al., 2008). It will take at least 2,000 to 4,000 units per day to reach the sufficiency range, with 6,400 units per day producing the most favorable results (Wagner et al., 2008; Holick, 2012). Furthermore, there may be as high as a 10-fold increase in vitamin D concentrations in breast milk with supplementation of 6,400 units vs. 400 units of vitamin D (Dawodu and Wagner, 2007). A daily intake of 6,400 units per day may seem high, but it is not. On a good day, getting enough sun exposure to create a light pink skin-tone response (in a white individual) will easily generate 10,000 to 20,000 units of vitamin D (Dawodu and Wagner, 2007). For the black individual, up to 10 times more sun exposure may be required to generate the same amount of vitamin D as a white individual (Wagner et al., 2008). Like who has *this* kind of time?

In the absence of adequate sun exposure, can you see how easy it is to become vitamin D deficient, particularly if you do not supplement with several thousand units of vitamin D per day? If you are black, you will <u>not</u> need 10 times the dose of a white individual, you will probably need the same dose, because vitamin D supplementation takes skin color completely out of the equation.

It only makes good common sense to supplement with an amount of vitamin D that will allow breast milk to be up to the task. A 6,000 IU daily dose of vitamin D will do this (plus the 400 IU from your prenatal). I say, give our kids the best start in life possible. Clearly, vitamin D sufficiency in the mother, passing <u>generous</u> amounts of vitamin D to the unborn and later to the hungry little newborn—the one who still needs "stuff" from Mom—is the only way to go. A formula will do (it *is* fortified with vitamin D), but "Mom" is clearly better. But is she up to the task? If you (or your physician) are a little nervous about 6,400 units of vitamin D per day, consider this:

> We note that the breastfeeding infants of these mothers have a substantially improved nutritional vitamin D status because of the transfer of vitamin D into mother's milk. Circulating 25(OH)D concentrations in the infants of mothers receiving the 4,000 IU/day dose increased into normal range after only 3 months of breastfeeding. (Hollis and Wagner, 2004)

Of course, always consult your physician before you supplement on your own. Blood testing seems, to me, to be the best starting point, and go from there, making sure that the mother has a respectable degree of vitamin D sufficiency and is receiving a level of supplementation tailored to meet her particular needs.

Imagine Your Baby not up to the task

Given recent discoveries that link vitamin D with the innate immune system, it is not unreasonable to predict that deficiencies during fetal development could have lasting sequelae [effects] on the child, not only in terms of bone mineralization, but also in terms of immune development that becomes the basis for later derangements seen with long-latency diseases such as multiple sclerosis, rheumatoid arthritis, diabetes, and certain cancers. **~Hamilton et al., 2010**

Interestingly, in later life, children of mothers with low vitamin D serum levels during pregnancy suffer more often from chronic diseases such as wheezing and asthma, schizophrenia, multiple sclerosis, type 1 diabetes mellitus and insulin resistance, suggesting intrauterine programming as a possible mechanism. **~Grundmann and von Versen-Höynck, 2011**

Vitamin D <u>sufficiency</u> is a gift from mother to child—both before and after birth . . . and is a gift that keeps on giving. Vitamin D <u>deficiency</u> is also a gift, one that may keep on giving and may bestow upon your child an increased risk of some very nasty things. Your baby, your child, may not be up to the task of defending him or herself against a variety of diseases that can have their beginnings in childhood (or earlier) and will continue harming them . . . for a lifetime. Type 1 diabetes and multiple sclerosis serve as examples. We will discuss all of this in an upcoming chapter entitled *Spare the Children*.

Nice!

I found the following guide on the internet, made just for the new mom. It covers so many useful things to know when it comes to the care of the newborn. Boy, there is a lot to this mommy business! Search for:

—Kaiser Permanente Healthy Beginnings - Issue 10

Perhaps the best way to find this guide is to go to the following website. From there you can click on Issue 10 and it will pop up in an instant. Print it out and put it to use. By the way, issues 1–9 are also available for this website at the click of a button. They are all great and will guide you through your entire pregnancy. Go to:

—Healthy Beginnings Newsletter
http://www.permanente.net/homepage/kaiser/pages/ f36294.html

Chapter 4
To be or not to be

It is well known that vitamin D deficiency is prevalent among pregnant women and pregnant women have significantly lower levels of 25(OH)D than nonpregnant control women. Approximately two in three pregnant women in the United States have suboptimal vitamin D status, with an even higher prevalence among black and Mexican-American women.
~Lerchbaum and Obermayer-Pietsch, 2012

In the United States, it is estimated that 50% of children aged 1–5 years and 70% of children aged 6–11 years are vitamin D deficient or insufficient. **~Holick, 2012**

Daily doses as high as 3,000 IU of vitamin D2 in premature infants, and 4,000 IU in older children, have been used to achieve 25(OH)D levels of 30 to 33 ng/mL without adverse effects. **~Huh and Gordon, 2008**

Because few foods naturally contain vitamin D, <u>it is essentially impossible</u> to satisfy their vitamin D requirement from dietary sources, unless a person eats oily fish 3–5 times a week. **~Holick, 2008, emphasis added**

Before we get into how easy it is for one to become vitamin D deficient, we need to learn how vitamin D sufficiency is achieved and how it is maintained. I will make this a relatively short chapter because there is nothing here that is all that complicated. Then, in the chapter to follow, we will take a look at what I call "The Red Flags of Vitamin D Deficiency." These are the indicators that strongly suggest that a mother-to-be is, or is likely to become, vitamin D deficient *and*

give birth to a vitamin D deficient baby. Of course, none of this is good.
It is bad. So, what is this thing called vitamin D deficiency? Why is it *so*
easy to come by?

Vitamin D deficiency 101

Vitamin D deficiency is a disease caused by sun deprivation.
~Holick, 2008

The lack of sufficient sun exposure *is* the cause of our epidemic of
vitamin D deficiency. **Nothing else**. And don't kid yourself, vitamin D
deficiency is a real epidemic (Holick, 2006a). And just like any other
epidemic, this one harms, this one kills. This one kills babies! And we
are of the belief that dietary vitamin D will stem the tide. We are *so*
mistaken.

> In comparison to sunlight, diet provides on average less than
> 10% of the body's vitamin D requirements in the best of
> circumstances. (Dawodu and Wagner, 2007)

While dietary sources of vitamin D are certainly helpful in
compensating for a lack of sun exposure, they are clearly not up to the
task (unless you are eating regularly of the fat of ocean fish or the
blubber of a savory walrus). This is why we supplement. This is why we
must supplement! Diet, generally, is <u>just</u> not enough. And for a variety
of reasons, we simply do not obtain enough sun exposure to meet our
needs.

The basics of vitamin D have now been covered. Sufficient sun
exposure equals vitamin D sufficiency. A deficiency of sun exposure
creates vitamin D deficiency. And diet (and your prenatal) just isn't
cutting it. Bottom line.

I don't want to disparage dietary sources of vitamin D—this is how we, as a society, squeak by. It is a safety net, keeping many from extremely low vitamin D levels. Sometimes, it is enough to make a big difference, keeping many in the sufficiency range. But, overall, it is simply not enough—particularly if you are in the baby-making business, a situation requiring higher amounts of vitamin D than usual (Berner et al., 2013). It gets worse. Those with darker skin are, once again, at special risk. According to one source, *"In the US, 45% of African American women have frank vitamin D deficiency as defined by a serum 25(OH)D concentration of less than 15 ng/ml."* (Dawodu and Wagner, 2007) Having darker skin (a natural sunscreen intended to protect the individual from a more sunlight-intense environment) clearly increases the disease burden in this segment of our population, including complications during pregnancy and adverse effects on their precious little ones. This is beyond sad. This is so preventable! More than any other, this population of individuals require a level of vitamin D supplementation that it never really receives. I am out to change this.

In our society—with our lifestyle of indoor living—we need to be promoting <u>effective</u> vitamin D supplementation <u>for everyone</u> in order to compensate for our lack of sun exposure. And of late, things seem to be getting worse, and the epidemic continues . . .

It's only getting easier!

In this national U.S. study, it was found that the average American spent 93% of their 24-hour day indoors. Since that time, air conditioning, computers, video games, and extensive television programming have become more readily available, increasing time spent indoors. Because of such changes in current lifestyles, humans are now more dependent on oral vitamin D supplementation than in our distant past. **~Wagner et al., 2008**

Subtly, our society has changed over the past few decades. Staying indoors is so much fun! We used to go outdoors to have fun, even to do our everyday chores. Then along came indoor plumbing, clothes dryers, TVs, video games, etc., and indoor living became a form of sunscreen. And it worked! We, as a society, have become more vitamin D deficient than in the past, both recent past and particularly so compared to our distant past, a time when we were hunger/gathers and outdoor bathers. Now we are just squeaking by. As a result, moms and babies—actually everyone!—are paying a price. We are the indoor people. We are the vitamin D deficient. We are also the sickly. The tragedy is, we know that supplementation is the answer to our lack of sun exposure, but we do it so poorly. And, the ones most affected are the ones who can do so little about it—the aliens that turn into babies and the babies that turn into children. Without adequate vitamin D supplementation, in the face of ever-decreasing sun exposure in our modern society, things are only going to get worse.

And this ain't gonna help!

Some dermatologists advise that people of all ages and ethnicities should avoid all direct exposure to sunlight and should always use sun protection when outdoors. **This message is not only unfortunate, it is misguided and has serious consequences,** *i.e., the risk of vitamin D deficiency.* ~**Holick, 2003, emphasis added**

Individuals are constantly told not to receive direct sun exposure or to wear sunscreen if they do. By following this advice, we are eliminating the initial step in an important endocrine system that can easily generate 10,000–20,000 IU/d vitamin D. ~**Hollis and Wagner, 2004**

The 30-year campaign of recommending abstinence from sun exposure has not decreased the incidence of non-melanoma skin cancer or melanoma, but it has promoted vitamin D deficiency. ~**Holick, 2008**

In our society, there is a war being waged. It is a war against sun exposure. And in this war, mistakes are being made. There is collateral damage. People could get hurt.

The dermatology community, as a whole, wants you to severely limit, even <u>eliminate,</u> sun exposure, or so it seems. They want to prevent skin cancer and put an end to epidemic of hideous wrinkles that has spread across the face of the land, and justifiably so. Theirs is a well-intentioned effort to help you; but, as the vitamin D research community will be eager to point out: avoiding sun exposure <u>and</u> the *religious* use of sunscreen will only intensify our epidemic of vitamin D deficiency (Holick, 2010). They will also eagerly point out that an individual can be sensible about sun exposure, can <u>easily</u> prevent sun burning—can even faithfully use sunscreen after an initial period of sun exposure—and still be able to generate all the vitamin D they need, for themselves and for their baby (supplementation may still be in order). They also believe that "sensible" sun exposure will actually help prevent skin cancer from occurring! (see Holick, 2006b; Holick, 2005; Bikle, 2009) So this should come as no surprise . . .

I hold the following opinion, and I am not alone: The OB/GYN community should join alongside those in the vitamin D research community in opposition of this *"unfortunate"* recommendation, the call for little or no sun exposure. The OB/GYN community, <u>above all others</u>, should warn you that, should you live your life primarily indoors, or should you religiously use sunscreen <u>before obtaining a reasonable period of sun exposure</u>, you may be jeopardizing your health and that of your baby, unless, of course, you supplement with vitamin D in relevant amounts. They should also be informing you that diet will not cut it and your prenatal vitamin is simply not up to the task. I can say this because the experts are saying this. Consider this:

Individuals are constantly told not to receive direct sun exposure or to wear sunscreen if they do. By following this advice, we are eliminating the initial step in an important endocrine system that can easily generate 10,000–20,000 IU/d vitamin D. How do we compensate for this? It is not likely with an intake of 400 IU/d vitamin D. Other confounding factors include dark skin pigmentation and northern latitudes, which inhibit cutaneous vitamin D3 production. We are rapidly becoming completely dependent on dietary supplementation as a means to ensure adequate vitamin D concentrations, and 400 IU/d is far from adequate. Second, maternal intake of 400 IU/d vitamin D does not elevate the nutritional status of mothers or nursing infants. This is indicated by the occurrence of hypovitaminosis D and rickets among breastfed infants. Maternal intake of 2,000 IU/d vitamin D elevates maternal 25(OH)D concentrations, but the amount passed on to nursing infants through the milk is still inadequate to elevate the infants' circulating 25(OH)D concentrations satisfactorily. Maternal intake of 4,000 IU/d increases maternal circulating concentrations to a degree that enough vitamin D enters the milk to produce significant effects on the infants' circulating 25(OH)D concentrations. (Hollis and Wagner, 2004)

Vitamin D insufficiency has been associated with a number of adverse pregnancy outcomes, and has been recognized as a public health concern. (Bener et al., 2013)

Now don't assume that all dermatologists want you to avoid sun exposure. Some have recognized that the benefits of "sensible" sun exposure may outweigh the risks. Here are the words of one:

Dermatologists and other physicians have to be aware that strict sun protection to prevent skin cancer may induce the severe health risk of vitamin D deficiency. To guarantee a sufficient vitamin D status, dermatological recommendations on sun protection and health campaigns for skin cancer prevention will have to be re-evaluated. There is no doubt that UV radiation is mutagenic and is the main reason for the development of non-melanoma skin cancer. Therefore, excessive sun exposure has to be avoided, particularly burning in childhood. To reach this goal, the use of sunscreens as well as the wearing of protective clothes and glasses is absolutely important. Additionally, sun exposure around midday should be avoided during the summer in most latitudes. However, the dermatological community has to recognize that there is convincing evidence that the protective effect of less intense solar radiation outweighs its mutagenic effect. In consequence, **many lives could be prolonged through careful exposure to sunlight or more safely, vitamin D supplementation, especially in non-summer months.** (Reichrath, 2007, emphasis added)

You don't have to go all nuts here when it comes to sun exposure. It has been reported that excessive sun exposure (think excessive sunbathing) may compromise one's folic acid status (Pérez-López, 2007). All I really want here is for you to be vitamin D sufficient. Use thoughtful, sensible sun exposure to accomplish this, unless contraindicated, and supplement, as needed, to make up for the lack of sun exposure. Restrict sun exposure if you must, but please maintain a vitamin D level that is sufficient, truly sufficient. And how you do this, generally, is with vitamin D supplementation in satisfactory amounts. Do what it takes to become vitamin D sufficient. That's all I ask. I am a reasonable man.

Sun exposure can be done right—even sunscreen can be done right, and should be generously applied after you first generate several thousand IU of vitamin D (takes about 10 to 15 minutes to do so if a reasonable amount of skin is exposed in the process). Go for a progressive tan. With this level of sun exposure, regularly achieved, you will likely be able to provide enough vitamin D to generously meet your needs and the needs of your unborn or newborn baby, late spring through fall. This 400 IU per day business is "woefully inadequate" (Hollis and Wagner, 2004). Vitamin D sufficiency is only accomplished by the regular production of thousands of units of vitamin D at a time, at least a couple of times a week, in the absence of relevant supplementation.   It is either adequate sun exposure or vitamin D supplementation in adequate amounts. You make the call. Someone is . . . well you know!

What is sensible sun exposure?

That is a good question. I will give you my take, based on what I have gleaned from the research literature.

Rule number 1: Don't get burned. This means that you do not, all of a sudden when Memorial Day rolls around, get in a boat and burn yourself to a crisp. No no no no no! You are ready for a limited amount of sun exposure at this point in the year—you haven't been outdoors all year! So this is what you do. First, make at least <u>some</u> vitamin D, then protect yourself with <u>generous</u> amounts of sunscreen. Wear a hat. Be at least partially clothed. Have some fun! Now it's summer time, we can get down to business. Attempt to go outdoors during mid-day, every day. Make it a habit of eating your lunch outside. If the sun is intense, limit exposure time. Under these circumstances, it only takes a little sun exposure to make plenty of vitamin D. Even after regular exposure to the sun, after a period of about 30 minutes, little if any vitamin D can be made by the recently exposed skin, so by all means follow up with all the sun protection you want. Please do! (Don't make me write a book on hideous wrinkles!) And keep this in mind: The more surface area of the body exposed, the less time you will need to intentionally create vitamin D. I'll be watching! Are you getting the idea? It is regular, frequent sun exposure, without the initial use of sunscreen—during the right time of day and during the right season of the year—that will likely create all the vitamin D you need (until winter rolls around). And you don't have to sunburn. This will only give sensible sun exposure a bad name (and harm you). And yes, *please* use sunscreen (please!) in your strategy to practice safe and sensible sun exposure. Some dermatologist (and author) is counting on you. This, I believe, is a sensible approach to the issue of sun exposure, vitamin D, and safety.

While it is clear that the lack of sun exposure leads to vitamin D deficiency, it is not all that clear that sun exposure will invariably lead to skin cancer (taking past sunburning events out to the equation). Consider this:

> The widespread concern about any direct sun exposure increasing the risk of the relatively benign and nonlethal squamous and basal cell cancers needs to be put into perspective. It is chronic excessive exposure to sunlight and sunburning experiences during childhood that increases risk of nonmelanoma skin cancer. Melanoma, one of the most feared cancers because of its ability to rapidly metastasize before it is obvious to either the patient or physician, has been branded as a sun-induced skin cancer.
>
> However, **most melanomas occur on the least sun-exposed areas**, and it has been reported that occupational exposure to sunlight decreases risk of melanoma. (Holick, 2006b, emphasis added)

Chapter 5
Red flags everywhere!

A reasonable practice seems to screen pregnant women at risk for hypovitaminosis D to ensure that their serum 25(OH)D level is higher than 30 ng/ml. Risk factors include reduced or inefficient sun exposure (i.e. season, latitude, lifestyle, non-caucasian ethnicity, concealing clothing) or pathological conditions (i.e., malabsorption, liver and kidney disease). **~Fanos et al., 2013**

Vitamin D deficiency during pregnancy is the origin for a host of future perils for the child. Some of this damage done by maternal Vitamin D deficiency becomes evident after many years. Therefore, prevention of vitamin D deficiency among pregnant women is essential. The current recommended supplementation amount of vitamin D is not sufficient during pregnancy. **~Kaushal and Magon, 2013**

Since vitamin D deficiency is caused by a lack of sun exposure (or the lack of adequate supplementation), it should come as no surprise that a good share of The Red Flags of Vitamin D Deficiency are related to patterns of living that restrict exposure to the sun. But there are other risk factors—some quite subtle—that can also lead to vitamin D deficiency. Feeling healthy may be the one most subtle! It can give you a false sense of security, settled in the belief that you are not at risk. I say, take the Red Flag Challenge! See how many Red Flags apply to you.

Location, location, location

Being born and living at lower latitudes [think more sun, more vitamin D] reduces the risk of developing type 1 diabetes by more than 10-fold and multiple sclerosis by more than 50%.   **~Holick, 2012**

Factors that limit or block the penetration of UVB radiation make it so easy to become vitamin D deficient. One factor is the latitude of residence. Living in a northern region of the country, say Boston, means that less UVB radiation will penetrate the atmosphere and be available for the generation of vitamin D than if one were to live, say, in the Bahamas. This all has to do the increased angle that occurs between sun light and atmosphere as latitude increases away from the equator, making it progressively more difficult for UVB radiation to penetrate (Holick, 2004). But there are no guarantees! Even if you live in sunny South Carolina, you can still be included among the vitamin D deficient. One team of investigators found nearly half of the study participants (pregnant women, aliens inside) to be vitamin D deficient, with an additional 37% considered to be vitamin D insufficient. (Hamilton et al., 2010).   Do the math. That leaves only 13% in the sufficiency range. **And we're talkin' sunny South Carolina!** Elsewhere, this same sort of thing has been found. *"It is surprising and disturbing to note that hypovitaminosis D is highly prevalent even in areas with adequate sunshine."* (Rathi and Rathi, 2011) **Not me!** I'm not surprised! No, not at all. It takes more than sun. It takes getting out into the sunshine, both causally and <u>intentionally</u> (and reasonably exposed), to achieve a level of vitamin D that is truly sufficient, unless, of course, one were to supplement adequately.

Many, many people live at a high latitude, live in an air-polluted region of the country, or live where the summer season is severely limited (think Alaska). These environmental circumstances restrict the amount of vitamin D that can be manufactured from sun exposure, and thereby increase one's risk of vitamin D deficiency (Lapillonne, 2010). Let's move on. I see more Red Flags ahead.

Ivory and Ebony

> *The renewed interest [in vitamin D] reflects the health attributes of vitamin D beyond metabolism and the widespread deficiency that affects all age groups but particularly those of dark pigmentation.* **~Wagner et al., 2008**

Race and ethnicity are clearly factors involved in the dynamic surrounding vitamin D deficiency. Compared to the light-skinned individual, those with dark skin are fundamentally more at risk of vitamin D deficiency. They are genetically inclined to tolerate, and require more sun exposure—more intense sun exposure!—in order to meet their needs for vitamin D. They have, built in, all the sunscreen they need (if dark enough), making sunburning less likely or next to impossible (Holick, 2004). It is this "natural" sunscreen that is the problem. In our society—in our corner of the globe—those who are black in any given locality are generally the ones most vitamin D deficient (Kaushal and Magon, 2013).

A black individual *will* need more sun exposure—up to 10 times more sun exposure—than an individual with light skin to manufacture an equivalent amount of vitamin D (Wagner et al., 2008). This is one reason why the African American community is so at risk of vitamin D deficiency. Add obesity, a condition affecting a *large* percent of our population (regardless of ethnicity), and the problem only intensifies. Then along come nice things followed by pregnancy. Now vitamin D deficiency becomes an invisible nightmare. In a study of black women in Pittsburg, nearly half of all pregnant black women were found vitamin D deficient, with only about 5% in the sufficiency range. (Bodnar et al., 2007c; Hewison and Adams, 2009). Some little alien is going to have a rough time of it and has a disproportionate chance of dying, all because maternal vitamin D sufficiency is harder to achieve in those with darker skin. And after birth indoor living will undoubtedly become a way of life for new little individual.   So the epidemic of vitamin D deficiency continues.

Shielded!

There is the claim that is purported by many in medicine that if one puts one's face and hands out the window for 15 minutes three times a week, such sunlight exposure will generate enough vitamin D to keep you in sufficient range. Unless you live at the equator, this is fallacious thinking. Sunlight exposure's effect on the body's synthesis of vitamin D depends on the surface area of the body exposed.   **~Wagner et al., 2008**

In the Middle East and Arab countries, time spent outdoors is severely limited and for cultural and religious reasons, the dress style of women outdoors prevents exposure of skin to sunlight.

In the US alone, Americans were found to spend an average of 93% of their time indoors.   **~Dawodu and Wagner, 2007**

Let's talk for a few moments about certain behaviors that limit the creation of vitamin D and lead to its deficiency. Being excessively clothed, staying indoors during the key period of the day when vitamin D can be synthesized, slapping on sunscreen before <u>any</u> sun exposure (in fear of skin cancer and hideous wrinkles), following cultural or religious practices that keep skin exposure to a minimum, and working practices that limit sunlight exposure—be it night-shift work followed by day sleeping, or seldom going outdoors on mid-day work breaks—are all practices that will restrict the creation of vitamin D . . . no matter where you live! You get the idea. It takes more that occasional or casual sun exposure to become vitamin D sufficient unless one duly compensates with adequate supplementation. It takes a deliberate effort to go outdoors during the time of day that vitamin D can be made to become vitamin D sufficient. By the way, sitting behind a window during the sunny part of the day will be of no help in this regard. Glass blocks the passage of UVB radiation. Now, are you beginning to see how easy it is to become vitamin D deficient no matter where you live?

Of course, I am very, very worried over this:

> In addition, the newborn infants of the veiled mothers showed an extremely high prevalence of vitamin D deficiency. (Dijkstra et al., 2007)

Everyone! Please go outdoors more often . . . into the sunshine. Expose enough of something to do a body good. Find a private area suitable for discrete sun exposure, if you must. Just get some sun on some skin, and do so on a regular basis. It has its rewards. Furthermore, I highly recommend that you take this book with you and read it outdoors. Bouncing sunlight off its pages and directly into your face can further improve your vitamin D status. (I'm sure that other books will do this, too, but probably not as well.)

This is a big deal!

> *Although a lowering of 25(OH)D concentrations with increasing BMI [body mass index] is worrisome for all adults, it is particularly concerning for pregnant women and their fetuses. Not only is poor in-utero and early-life vitamin D status related to long-term negative effects of the offspring, but maternal vitamin D deficiency may also increase the risk of adverse pregnancy outcomes.* ~Bodnar et al., 2007b

Your body weight, if excessive, is one big Red Flag. The reason is two-fold. Your skin is a little thicker, impeding the penetration of UVB radiation, the wavelength of light that makes vitamin D from cholesterol (Cantor, 2008). On top of that, any vitamin D that you make or take will very likely be sequestered in your fat reserves (Holick, 2004a). You are storing fat for a rainy day. You are also storing vitamin D for a rainy day.

You have become a storage depot of epic proportions. This makes vitamin D less available to meet your present needs (Holick, 2004a). I sure hope you are supplementing in a relevant amounts! Your doctor will advise (I hope). Remind him or her that you are, sadly, an indoor person. Follow up with a reminder that, even when outdoors and in the sun, you are only able to manufacture only about half the amount for vitamin D that those annoying little skinny people who are able to manufacture tons of vitamin D at the drop of a hat (Wortsman et al., 2000).

In our society, we really do have a **big** problem on our hands. It is obesity. And it definitely intensifies our epidemic of vitamin D deficiency.

Nearly one third of all U.S. adults are categorized as obese. (Parikh et al., 2004)

Obesity is often associated with vitamin D deficiency. It is now recognized that, whether vitamin D is ingested or obtained from exposure to sunlight, it is efficiently deposited in the large body fat stores and is not bioavailable. This is probably the reason that obese persons are chronically vitamin D deficient. (Holick, 2004b)

And, of course, an obese mother, typically, will only have limited amounts of vitamin D to share with the one who is developing inside. Vitamin D deficiency "imposed" in this matter is, undoubtedly, one of the reasons that the babies of obese mothers have more than their fair share of health problems.

Say it isn't so!

I'm so worried about you, as it is. And now you are telling me that you are dealing with some hideous medical condition? *What am I going to do with you?!!* I know! I'll give you some friendly advice.

If you have Crohn's disease or some kind of diabolical fat malabsorption syndrome like cystic fibrosis or celiac disease, or if you have undergone stomach surgery or gastric bypass surgery in the past, you are one big walking, talking Red Flag (Holick, 2006; Zhang and Naughton, 2010). No one wants to be you (although they may want to mate with you). You *will* need special attention with respect to vitamin D. You are <u>automatically</u> at high risk of deficiency. And when pregnant or nursing, your baby is, <u>automatically</u>, at high risk of vitamin D deficiency.

Good drug, bad drug

Talk with your doctor if you are pregnant and you have taken any medication or are thinking of taking any medication. This includes prescription and over-the-counter medications, as well as dietary or herbal products. **~CDC, 2013**

Phenobarbital, phenytoin, carbamazepine (all anticonvulsants), rifampicin (an antibiotic)—all are drugs that increase the catabolism (consumption, breakdown) of vitamin D (Zhang and Naughton, 2010). Steroids and certain drugs used in the treatment of cancer may also contribute to vitamin D deficiency (Wortsman et al., 2000; Fakih et al., 2009). Plaquenil, a drug used to treat both lupus (Huisman et al., 2001) and rheumatoid arthritis (*Web*MD, 2012) may also lower vitamin D levels (Barnes and Bucknall 2004). Ask your physician if other medications you are taking promote vitamin D deficiency—you need to be reviewing all your meds anyway, as some can really harm your baby. Run through the list! Include over-the-counter meds, herbs, even supplements, too.

Why did you ever start?

Various factors such as nutrition, alcohol and caffeine consumption, the sun exposure, skin pigmentation, obesity, physical activity, clothing and

seasonal variation can affect vitamin D status and bone metabolism during
pregnancy.

Cigarette smoke exposure during pregnancy has effects on pregnancy
such as increased spontaneous abortion, low birth weight, placenta
detachment, premature rupture of membranes, intrauterine growth
restriction and vaginal bleeding. **~Banihossein et al., 2013**

You know the drill. If you are a smoker, you need to stop. **Now!**
You are pregnant and have no other choice. But what about alcohol?

It has long been known that excessive alcohol consumption has
a negative impact on vitamin D status. Chronic alcoholism results in
disturbed vitamin D metabolism and chronic alcoholics usually have
low levels of vitamin D. (Lee, 2012, paraphrased)

You know the drill. You know what to do. Actually, what not to do.
But what about caffeine?

Caffeine may actually raise vitamin D levels! (Al-Othman et al.,
2012) But this worries me. Caffeine may interfere with the conversion
of circulating form of vitamin D into the "active" form (Al-Othman et al.,
2012). This may lead to a deficiency of the active form of vitamin D,
negatively affecting both you and your baby. Ask your physician what
he or she thinks. Caffeine should probably be limited during pregnancy,
regardless of any effect it has on the vitamin D status of the mother-to-
be and that of the unborn.

Of course, addictive substances create addicted little aliens, so be
careful out there. Some dangers seem so innocent. The harm caused
can be so great. And you're not going to want to hear this:

Marijuana can affect fetal and infant development and may
cause miscarriage. Although the effects of marijuana on an unborn
baby are still unknown, studies have indicated that prenatal
marijuana use is linked to premature births, small birth size, difficult
or long labor and an increase in newborn jitteriness.

Marijuana smoked by a pregnant woman remains in the baby's fat cells for seven to 30 days. Smoking marijuana can affect the amount of oxygen and nutrients the baby receives, which may affect growth. **Marijuana is never safe during pregnancy and it can harm the baby at any stage.** In addition, marijuana can have long-term effects on infants and children, such as having trouble paying attention or learning to read. (UCSF Medical Center, 2002–2014, emphasis added)

Dieting to the extreme

Dietary factors like very low calcium intake and high fiber diet may deplete vitamin D stores. ~**Rathi and Rathi, 2011**

There are other dietary issues to consider, all potentially impacting one's vitamin D status. For example, avoiding milk or limiting milk consumption will affect one's vitamin D status. The same applies to avoiding or limiting other fortified foods, like orange juice. Both milk and oranges are good sources of vitamin D because we make them good sources of vitamin D. You can squeak by better when both are regularly consumed. But I see another problem.

Vegetarianism, allowing eggs and milk, is not a big concern with respect to the risk of vitamin D deficiency, generally. A vegan diet? Now that's an area of concern! (Unless one obtains plenty of sunshine or supplements in satisfactory amounts). (see Misra et al., 2008; Craig, 2009) The vegan will need to supplement with D2 (a vegetarian source of vitamin D) if D3 (the vitamin D of animal origin) is objectionable. Sunshine is, of course, more necessary than ever if you are a vegan. Winter, of course, would be a big problem for the vegan, particularly if pregnant. Better supplement! Some little someone is counting on you.

While not necessarily diets, eating disorders naturally lead to vitamin deficiencies. If an eating disorder is a part of your life, make sure your physician is well aware. Get some help. And get tested for vitamin D deficiency. You may also be at increased risk for a B12 deficiency. Get tested for this, as well. The vegetarian and the vegan should also be tested for B12 deficiency before and during pregnancy, in my opinion.

How you feelin' hun?

Upper respiratory tract infections (colds) and influenza (flu) are more frequent when vitamin D intake and stores are at their lowest (Holick, 2010). If you are one who catches colds easily, comes down with the flu at the drop of a hat, consider that vitamin D deficiency may be the reason. And, may I ask, if you suffer from winter depression, more formally called seasonal affective disorder (SAD)—actually, any form of mental illness—get tested for vitamin D deficiency. (see Gracious et al., 2012) It is very common for vitamin D deficiency to be associated with disorders affecting the brain. Chances are you will be found deficient.

And, may I add. If you feel tired all the time, and have muscle aches and pains, it is very likely you are vitamin D deficient (Holick, 2004b; Holick, 2007). Here's a test, one that is free: Using your fingers, place a moderate amount of pressure on your breast bone. If this causes pain, you are very likely to be, or have been, vitamin D deficient for an extended period of time (Holick, 2007). The pain comes from improper mineralization of the outer layer of bone due to chronic vitamin D deficiency.

Last flag standing

I almost failed to mention this: If you are reading this book, and even if you are not reading this book, you are probably vitamin D deficient. *Existing* is a risk factor for vitamin D deficiency and should be considered to be big a Red Flag.

Gone too far

Occasionally vitamin D deficiency in an infant or child becomes a very big deal, sometimes life threatening! <u>Severe</u> vitamin D deficiency (and we're talkin' *severe*) can cause seizures (Wallis, 2008). The heart can also fail (Carlton-Conway et al., 2004). Such adverse effects as these are likely to occur <u>only</u> if vitamin D deficiency is extreme. Perhaps a child may develop muscle aches and pain should vitamin D deficiency persist over a long period of time (Whyman et al., 2010). Although such expressions of vitamin D deficiency are rare, the physician (and the mother or father) should be aware that vitamin D deficiency may be behind other less "classical" expressions, such as a severe and unexplained illness in an infant or a child. It may be behind what is called failure to thrive (Schmalz et al., 2009). And, it could be mistaken for child abuse.

This is so sad. A loving parent, a sick infant or child, a physical examination followed by an x-ray or two, the finding of healed arm or rib fractures or other signs that suggest physical abuse, and suspicions are raised. Eyebrows are lifted. Sometimes babies are taken away from their parents . . . all due to vitamin D deficiency, mistakenly thought to be abuse or neglect. (see Keller and Barns, 2008; Chesney, 2008; Paterson, 2009)

Too much of a good thing

Vitamin D *can* be taken in excess. Rarely, one will find a case of vitamin D toxicity—practically never from sun exposure (Holick, 2004a) but possibly by accident or by increased sensitivity. Don't worry. It is doubtful that a daily dose of 6,400 units of vitamin D per day will cause toxicity in the average person. Indeed, doses of upwards to **100,000, yes 100,000**, units per day have been given to pregnant women under special circumstances with <u>no</u> adverse effects observed in mother or infant (Dror and Allen, 2010). But don't even think of trying this on your own! High dose (e.g., 100,000 IU) vitamin D is reserved for <u>very</u> unusual medical situations.

Surprisingly, even a little vitamin D supplementation may be too much for some individuals, making vitamin D supplementation inappropriate or to be conducted using extreme caution. The doctor will explain (he knows a lot of big words):

> Reported side effects of vitamin D include nausea, vomiting, headache, metallic taste, vascular or nephrocalcinosis, and pancreatitis.Reported contraindications to vitamin D include hypercalcemia in sarcoidosis; metastatic bone disease; other granulomatous diseases such as tuberculosis and Crohn's disease (active phase) that have a disordered vitamin D metabolism in activated macrophages; and Williams syndrome (infantile hypercalcemia). (Schwalfenberg, 2007)

The above quotation reinforces my belief that it is best to supplement with vitamin D under medical supervision. Testing, of course, is how we know if we are on track, getting too much, or not getting enough.

More thoughts about B12

I made mention of the importance of B12 before, but I need to add more.

Like vitamin D, B12 is a very important vitamin (probably a hormone, as well). Its deficiency can lead to neurological problems that may never go away. Vegetarians—especially vegans—are at increased risk of B12 deficiency. If pregnant or nursing, *someone* may not get their fair share. Supplementation may be in order for both mother and baby. The Red Flags that raise the risk of B12 deficiency in mom include Crohn's disease, celiac disease, a certain type of anemia called pernicious anemia, Graves' disease, and lupus. Excessive alcohol consumption and long-term use of acid-reducing drugs can also lead to vitamin B12 deficiency. (*Web*MD, 2012)

Chapter 6
Spare the children

Vitamin D deficiency during pregnancy has been linked with a number of serious short- and long-term health problems in offspring, including impaired growth, skeletal problems, type 1 diabetes, asthma, and schizophrenia. **~Bodnar et al., 2007a**

In the United States, it is **estimated that 50% of Children 1–5 years and 70% of children age 6–11 years are vitamin D deficient or insufficient.** *This has potentially serious consequences.* **~Holick, 2012, emphasis added**

Pediatricians should have a low threshold for screening for vitamin D deficiency in the presence of nonspecific symptoms such as poor growth, gross motor delays, and unusual irritability. **~Misra et al., 2008**

Even infants born to vitamin D replete [sufficient] mothers become vitamin D deficient after 8 weeks if not supplemented by vitamin D, while an unsupplemented infant born to a vitamin D deficient mother will reach a state of deficiency more quickly than an infant whose mother was replete during pregnancy. **~Dawodu and Wagner, 2007**

Regular and sensible sun exposure during the months of the year when vitamin D production is promoted is still the most physiologic way to prevent vitamin D deficiency in infants and children. **~Holick, 2006**

I want to spare babies. I want to spare children. I have nothing better to do. **There *is* nothing better to do!** This is why I wrote a certain little book on mommies, babies, and vitamin D . . . just for you. And I hate to be the one to have to tell you this (again), but there a multitude of diseases lying in wait, diseases that cannot wait to claim another victim. It could be your child! Vitamin D deficiency will allow them to do this, and claim with greater ease. I see so much trouble ahead, but less trouble ahead if you make sure that both you and your little one(s) become and remain vitamin D sufficient. Some favorite author is counting on you.

So, what are the diseases that await the child who was, who is, and who remains vitamin D deficient? We'll run through the big ones, one by one—and these are diseases that can be prevented, in good measure, if vitamin D is in adequate supply. We'll start first with the skeletal system.

Bone deformity and compromise

Rickets is an extreme form of vitamin D deficiency and represents the tip of the iceberg. ~**Rathi and Rathi, 2011**

Adequate vitamin D concentrations during pregnancy help ensure appropriate maternal and fetal calcium homeostasis [appropriateness] and bone metabolism. Consequently, vitamin D deficiency during pregnancy has been associated with impaired fetal skeletal formation causing infant rickets and reduced bone mass. ~**Zhao et al., 2012**

Interestingly, vitamin D deficiency during pregnancy is also associated with risks of health problems later in childhood, including improper bone development at 9 years of age, asthma, dental cavities, schizophrenia, and type 1 diabetes. ~**Kaushal and Magon, 2013**

A lack of vitamin D during pregnancy results in poor fetal and infant bone mineralization that may persist into later life. ~**Shand et al., 2010**

Why do I feel the need to comment at all? The quotations above tell the story. And Medicine is well aware of the relationship between vitamin D and bone integrity! After all, it was the attention paid to vitamin D deficiency and rickets that piqued our interest in vitamin D in the first place. We know this part of the story so very well. Or do we?

Rickets represents an extreme expression of vitamin D deficiency. It is characterized by bowed legs, pain, muscle weakness, bones that break with ease, growth retardation, and increased susceptibility to infections. We vanquished this disease years ago, or so we thought. It has, unfortunately, made a comeback (Holick, 2006; Bodnar et al., 2007c). It can pop up, here and there, and can be easily spotted by those who are on their toes. It is a world-wide problem, occurring even in the good ol' USA, a large share occurring in black babies who are exclusively breast fed (Bodnar et al., 2007c).

But even if the bones of an infant or child appear strong and reasonably well developed, we may still have a big problem on our hands. It certainly seems that bones believe they are the most important part of the body and will grab all the vitamin D they can get a hold of in an effort to fulfill their needs, leaving less available for other important tasks. This sort of thing can happen before birth and this sort of thing can happen after birth when supplies of vitamin D are insufficient. Fortunately, the bones can't grab it all, so there is at least some vitamin D floating around somewhere to meet the needs of other tissues and cells, but generally not enough. And although rickets may be avoided when the bones taking the lion's share of available vitamin D, there can still be a problem with the integrity of the bones when vitamin D levels remain low during development. This can lead osteoporosis and fractures later in life (Holick, 2006).

What is quite surprising is that we can prevent rickets all day long, all the while we allow a baby or a child to remain vitamin D deficient all day long, day after day after day after day after day. Some who feel that the absence of rickets is a sign that vitamin D must be in adequate supply and recommend supplementing with, basically, the amount of vitamin D it takes to prevent this disease (200 to 400 IU/day) are missing a golden opportunity to play a part in preventing a number of diseases well worth preventing. Type 1 diabetes is well worth preventing.

Type 1 diabetes

Vitamin D deficiency in utero and during the first year of life has also been linked to increased risk of type 1 diabetes. 1,25(OH)$_2$D affects the immune system, and, as pancreatic islet β cell have a VDR, it also stimulates insulin secretion. Thus, hypovitaminosis D in children may increase their risk not only of type 2 diabetes but also insulin resistance and islet β cell dysfunction. **~Holick, 2006**

Astonishingly, they found that children who received vitamin D supplementation at the recommended 2,000 IU/d had **reduced the risk of developing diabetes type 1 by 80%.** **~Holick, 2002, emphasis added**

In the United States approximately 15,000 children every year are diagnosed with type 1 diabetes. That's over 40 kids per day! What if just one could be spared? What if many could be spared? What if vitamin D could make all the difference in the world?

Type 1 diabetes results from an autoimmune destruction of the insulin producing β cells of the pancreas (Harris, 2005). And this disease process can begin very early, within months after birth (Harris, 2005; Knip et al., 2005). Insulin is the hormone that allows us to use glucose as a fuel. Cells starve when glucose is not in adequate supply. In the past, type 1 diabetes was rapidly fatal. Then along came insulin as a medication, and we began to tame this disease. But I would rather prevent this disease. It is still one very bad boy. Alarmingly, the death rate is **seven times** the death rate of those who do not have type 1 diabetes. And, *"Women with type 1 diabetes are **13 times** more likely to die [prematurely from disease] than women who did not have diabetes."* (source: American Diabetes Association, 2010, emphasis added) It certainly worth preventing, this disease we call type 1 diabetes.

Due to its positive effects of the immune system, along with its beneficial effects on the health of the insulin producing β cells themselves, vitamin D had been shown to be able to prevent this disease from taking hold, and has done so in a very dramatic way.

In a much-celebrated study, 10,366 Finnish children were followed for a period of 30 years. Surprisingly, those who received 2,000 units of vitamin D per day, a recommendation of the day, *"were 80% less likely to develop type 1 diabetes."* (Walker and Modlin, 2009; Holick, 2006) And what is today's recommendation for vitamin D in the first year of life? A silly 400, perhaps 600 IU per day (Hollis et al., 2011). Good grief! This is the dose we squeak by with (if we're lucky), not the dose we prevent type 1 diabetes with (see Harris, 2005). I see trouble ahead—excuse me while I go and bang my head against the wall.

> Vitamin D deficiency in pregnancy probably increases the incidence of autoimmune diseases, such as type 1 diabetes, in genetically predisposed individuals

> A major clinical lesson that can be drawn at this moment is that avoidance of vitamin D deficiency is essential for β-cell function, and might contribute to protection against type 1 diabetes in later life. (Mathieu and Badenhoop, 2005)

It seems like we could save some kids from type 1 diabetes if we really wanted to.

> Vitamin D supplementation in infancy seems to exert a strong protective effect against the autoimmune disease type I diabetes, and vitamin D levels in early childhood could also have an impact on the risk of MS. (Munger et al., 2006)

Multiple Sclerosis

The prevalence of MS is nearly zero close to the equator and is markedly increased in regions of more northern latitudes. **~Zittermann, 2003**

Early sun avoidance seems to precede the diagnosis of multiple sclerosis (MS). This protective effect is independent of genetic susceptibility to MS. **~Islam et al., 2007, emphasis added**

Early life sunlight exposure and dietary vitamin D supplementation diminish the risk of MS. **~Chaudhuri, 2005**

*Living above the 35° latitude [above Los Angeles or Atlanta, for example] for the first 10 years of life imprints on a child for the rest of his or her life a **100% increased risk** [double the risk] of developing multiple sclerosis no matter where they live thereafter.* **~Holick** 2006, **emphasis added**

Another study checked the vitamin D intake in more than 187,000 women from two separate cohorts (study groups) . . . and found a 40% reduction in the risk of multiple sclerosis among women who used supplemental vitamin D. **~Arnson et al., 2007**

Mice that were pretreated with 1,25(OHO)$_2$D3 before they were injected with myelin to induce a multiple-sclerosis like disease were immune from it. **~Holick, 2005**

Multiple sclerosis (MS) is a disease that effects about 2.5 million people worldwide. Approximately, 200 Americans receive this diagnosis each and every week (source: multiplesclerosis.net). I have placed this disease on my *Let-Somebody-Else-Get-This-One-And-Not-Me* list, right near the top. An individual with multiple sclerosis may look normal on the outside, but inside . . . another story. The person's immune system has launched a progressive attack on the insulation (myelin sheath) that covers the nerves in the brain and spinal cord, the nerves involved become damaged and messages simply do not get through. The spirit is willing, but the flesh is weak. Bad disease! And so related to a lack of sunlight exposure that it is crazy! *Crazy!*

The sad thing is that it can have its foundation during fetal development, as early as the first trimester (Staples et al., 2010). We typically assume that this is an adult-onset disease. But kids get this disease, too. Approximately, 8,000 to 10,000 children in the US have MS at the top of their list of problems to deal with . . . for life (*Web*MD, 2013). And, although the disease may have its beginnings during gestation (some little somebody was counting on mom), sun exposure later in life (think more vitamin D) could make all the difference in the world.

One study of identical twins found that "*the twin who spent more time suntanning in comparison with the co-twin*" had a "*significantly*" lower risk of MS (Islam et al., 2007). This group of investigators, Islam et al, studied one population group and discovered that "*2 to 3 hours of youthful sun exposure on average per week were found to have nearly a 60% reduction of MS risk.*" (Islam et al., 2007) And we know what sunshine exposure means. It means an increased level of vitamin D (and a nice, attractive tan).

I could go on and on regarding the relationship between sunshine, vitamin D and MS risk, but we must hurry things along. We have another dreadful disease to prevent.

Crohn's disease (CD)

Living at higher latitude and being prone to vitamin D deficiency increases the risk of several autoimmune disease including type 1 diabetes and Crohn's disease. **~Holick, 2006**

It appears that CD incidence is higher in geographical areas with a low sunshine exposure than in areas with high or medium sunshine exposure. **~Nerich et al., 2011**

Investigators . . . found that vitamin D-sufficient women were 62% less likely to be diagnosed with CD during a 22-year period compared with those deemed sufficient. **~Medscape Medical News, 2012**

So, here we have yet another disease on our hands that may be prevented, to a significant degree, by sun exposure and vitamin D sufficiency. And this is one very nasty disease. It can cause abdominal pain, intestinal ulcerations and bleeding, diarrhea galore, and any number of other disturbing complications (you don't want to know). It appears to be an autoimmune attack on the bowel, when, in fact, it is a disease of impaired defense against bacteria (Kelsall, 2008; Yamamoto-Furusho and Korzenik, 2006). And, as we have learned, one role for vitamin D is for defense against bacterial invasion (Liu et al., 2009; Gombart, 2009). The immune cells can destroy more effectively when vitamin D is in adequate supply. Crohn's disease can make life very difficult and create the need for multiple surgical interventions. You don't want this disease. You don't want your child to have this disease. **You don't want <u>anyone</u> to have this disease!** Listen up!

In adults, *"Higher predicted levels of 25(OH)D significantly reduced the risk for incident CD."* (Ananthakrishnan et al., 2012) In the study just quoted, it was estimated that for every 100 IU of vitamin D per day, there was a 7% reduction in the incidence of Crohn's disease (Ananthakrishnan et al., 2012). I suspect that, if vitamin D sufficiency will prevent Crohn's in adults, it will do the same in children. Apparently, 1 out of every 5 individuals with this disease is, sadly, a child (Children's Hospital of Wisconsin, 2013). And since there are approximately 500,000 individuals in the US suffering from Crohn's, there are approximately 100,000 kids in the US suffering from this disease. All this Crohn's! All this suffering! *This* has to stop! And I am doing something about it. I'll tell you more in the gray box at the end of this chapter.

There is another angle for us to consider here, related to vitamin D deficiency and the risk of childhood Crohn's—one of those "one thing leads to another" . . . things.

For a variety of medical reasons, antibiotic use is common in childhood (Hviid et al.., 2011). Preemies often need antibiotics to deal with infections acquired in the hospital setting or they will not survive. By the way, preemies are often vitamin D deficient at birth, and preemies may be preemies due to vitamin D deficiency during gestation (see chapter 2). On occasion, a term baby will need an antibiotic. And later in life, here come the sinus infections, the ear infections, and the pneumonias that occur more frequently in those who are deficient in vitamin D. Understandably, we turn to antibiotics to help us solve the problem at hand, and a lot of antibiotics *are* given to our kids as they stumble through life, many times unnecessarily. Unfortuinately, with antibiotic use, we have an unanticipated pathway leading directly to childhood Crohn's.

One group of investigators noticed a strong association between antibiotic use and Crohn's, with the disease occurring in as little as 3 months following several courses of antibiotics (Hviid et al., 2011).

Another group determined that inflammatory bowel disease, Crohn's included, was nearly 3 times more likely if antibiotics were used within the first year of life (Shaw et al., 2010).

And, *"Hildebrand et al. found that individuals diagnosed with pneumonia before 5 years of age were at almost three-fold the odds of developing pediatric CD, compared to those with no recorded pneumonia diagnosis,"* antibiotic use presumed (Shaw et at., 2010).

So, as you can see, vitamin D deficiency . . . leading to infections . . . leading to antibiotic use . . . can lead to Crohn's disease in an innocent little child . . . and a life is forever changed.

We'd better move on, I see more trouble ahead. But then again, I am always seeing more trouble ahead. *Trouble!*

Infectious disease

Infants and children appear to be more susceptible to viral rather than bacterial infections. **~Walker and Modlin, 2009**

Vitamin D deficiency seems to be a risk factor for severe respiratory infection in children <5 years of age. **~Laaksi et al., 2010**

Furthermore, black children continue to have twice the pneumonia mortality of white children. **~Cannell et al., 2011**

Infections occur more frequently in the vitamin D deficient, particularly upper respiratory infection. This is fairly obvious. All that sniffling! All that snot! Someone needs to do something, and fast! Too bad, vitamin D deficiency in an infant and in a child is so very, very common. Someone could get sick.

At birth, if the cord blood is tested and the baby is found to be vitamin D deficient, he or she is more likely to have a respiratory infection within the following 3 months (Camargo Jr. et al., 2011). Why am I not surprised? With less vitamin D on board, the baby's immune system is simply not up to the task (Camargo Jr. et al., 2007). Vitamin D deficiency in a baby is the gift of immunodeficiency. It is the gift of vulnerability. But it doesn't have to be that way. We can lessen the risk.

As early as birth a child is often deficient in vitamin D, which may not only affect their bone metabolism but also modulate their immune function, contributing to the increased susceptibility to many infections seen early in life. (Battersby et al., 2012)

Need I say more? Probably.

Asthma

Epidemological evidence suggests that there is a worldwide epidemic of vitamin D deficiency, and a lack of vitamin D has been linked to increased incidence of asthma and increased severity of asthma in children.
~Bener et al., 2012

Asthma is the most common chronic disease in childhood (Bener et al., 2012; Litonjua, 2009). If a child wheezes before 3 years of age, he or she is 10 times more likely to have asthma by age 6 (Camargo Jr. et al., 2007). This disease is annoying to say the least. It can also take a child's life. For example, 185 US children died from asthma in 2007 (source: American Academy of Allergy Asthma & Immunology, 2014). That is at least 185 US children too many. The association between vitamin D deficiency during pregnancy and lactation and childhood asthma in the offspring is considered to be strong (Camargo Jr. et al., 2007; Bener et al., 2012). And, of course, it makes sense. During fetal development, *"vitamin D appears to play a role in immune system and lung development."* (Lange et al., 2009).

Let's take a moment to catch our breath before we take a look at the impact vitamin D deficiency has on the developing mind.

Who would have thought?

The central nervous system is increasingly being recognized as a target organ for vitamin D via its wide-ranging steroid hormone effects and via the induction of various proteins such as nerve growth factor.
~McGrath, 1999

Our results indicate that gestational vitamin D deficiency has profound effects on the developing brain, including changes in volume, shape, cell proliferation and growth factor expression. **~Eyles et al., 2003**

Thus far, we have paid little attention to the most important part of the child, the child's brain—I guess there were too many other important considerations we needed to take a look at first. But when it comes to making a baby, a nice brain, in good working order, is really what we are after. Cuteness and chubby little cheeks do not even come close.

Proper brain development, naturally, begins in the womb. And it continues after birth—actually *forever!*—that is, until the curtain comes down. There is quite a vitamin D story here! Let's take a look.

Schizophrenia

In utero or early life vitamin D deficiency has been linked to an increased risk of type 1 diabetes, asthma, and schizophrenia. **~Bodnar et al., 2007c**

The absence of vitamin D supplementation during infancy was associated with an increased risk of schizophrenia. **~McGrath et al., 2004**

Remember the 10,366 Finnish children who were found to have an 80% less chance of contracting type 1 diabetes if they were supplemented with 2,000 units of vitamin D per day during their first year of life? Well, someone else remembered this and decided to see if the risk of schizophrenia was also reduced in this same group of individuals. Surprisingly, the risk was reduced by **77%** in the male subjects, in those who received vitamin D supplementation (McGrath et al., 2004). It is unclear as to why a statistic was not generated in the female subjects, as no female in the entire study population came down with schizophrenia later in life. Some believe it is the female hormones that offer increased protection against schizophrenia, offsetting the negative effects of hypovitaminosis D (Cannell, 2008). For once, the ladies catch a break.

Although it is relatively common, you may not know what schizophrenia is. Schizophrenia is a disease characterized by disturbed thought processes and an insufficient grasp on reality. It can be mild or it can be devastating. It can be your worst nightmare! So much heartache for so many moms. Experimentally, making an animal vitamin D deficient during gestation causes brain malformation and dysfunction, without fail (Eyles et al., 2003; Eyles et al., 2009). When the brain is analyzed in patients with schizophrenia, both before and after death, the brain is incorrectly formed and appears to have functional abnormalities as well—similar to what is seen in studies on animals (Féron et al., 2005; Eyles et al., 2003; Kiraly et al., 2006; McCann and Ames, 2008). Experimentally and in real life, there is a considerable amount of evidence to indicate that low vitamin D availability during gestation is a recipe for disaster. And the brain can become a disaster area.

Perhaps the strongest evidence that vitamin D deficiency during gestation increases the risk of schizophrenia comes from immigration studies. It has been observed a number of times and in a number of places that those with dark skin who migrate from a sunny region to a region with lower levels of UVB intensity have substantial increase in the incidence of schizophrenia in the offspring (Dealberto, 2006; McGrath, 1999). Accordingly;

> Immigrant status is an important environmental risk factor not only for schizophrenia but also for other psychoses.

> European researchers have observed that **schizophrenia is 3 times more frequent** in immigrants than in native-born subjects. This increased risk is even higher in dark-skinned immigrants, and the second generation is more affected than the first. (Dealberto, 2006, emphasis added)

Let's keep this simple. Vitamin D is a hormone involved in the structural development of the brain and is necessary for proper brain activity. If vitamin D supplies are low, the brain will face challenges. It may become both structurally and/or functionally compromised and simply not have what it takes to hold tightly onto reality. That's about all you need to know for the moment. But go ahead and add this:

> Unfortunately, it appears that the effects of gestational vitamin D deficiency may result in long-term, or even permanent, alterations in the brain of the offspring that cannot be overcome by postnatal vitamin D supplementation. (Levenson and Figuerôa, 2008)

I think it's is best to be vitamin D sufficient during pregnancy. Some little brain is . . . well you know.

Depression

> *Vitamin D deficiency has been linked to an increased incidence of schizophrenia and depression. Maintaining vitamin D sufficiency in utero and during early life, to satisfy the vitamin D receptor transcriptional activity in the brain, may be important for brain development as well as for maintenance of mental function later in life.* **~Holick, 2007**

> ***It is clear that disrupting prenatal vitamin D can have significant effects on the developing brain with adverse consequences later in life.*** **~Markham and Koenig, 2011, emphasis added**

Depression is not just reserved for those who seem to have everything but for some reason just cannot find happiness. Kids also become depressed, and for a variety of reasons. And I don't mean the prolonged despondency you feel when your parents will not allow you to keep a pony in your bedroom. (I still have not fully recovered from this experience.) No, I'm talking about a heaviness that lingers in the mind, weighs down a child, and deprives the child of experiencing the joy of living. Depression is a shadow hovering over a life. Self-esteem, one of the greatest assets in life, takes a big hit. Behavior problems in childhood can emerge. Vitamin D deficiency could be a factor! Don't let it happen.

The surprising thing about depression is the fact that it can manifest itself in so many different ways. *"The symptoms of depression in children vary. It is often undiagnosed and untreated because they are passed off as normal emotional and psychological changes that occur during growth."* (WebMD, 2012) Symptoms of depression in children can include difficulty concentrating, social withdrawal, irritability, mood swings, and thoughts of suicide—another one of your worst nightmares. Incidentally, suicide attempts apparently occur more frequently during spring, the season of the year when vitamin D levels are at their lowest (Tariq et al., 2011). Hmm. I find this depressing.

I could locate only a few studies that report an association between low vitamin D and depression in children. In one study the investigators noticed a delayed effect of 9.8 years between low vitamin D levels and the onset of childhood depression (Tolppanen et al., 2012a). In other words, they didn't find anything of real value. But others have.

In another study, a group of 54 adolescents suffering from depression were tested for vitamin D deficiency, and, of course, were found to be, for lack of a better word, deficient (Högberg et al., 2012). On average, their vitamin D level in was 16.4 ng/ml (pretty low), with 6 individuals presenting with a vitamin D level of 10 ng/ml (very low). The intention of this study was to identify a group of depressed adolescents and supplement them with vitamin D to see if depressive symptoms would improve. They did. After 4,000 IU of vitamin D daily for 1 month, followed by 2,000 IU for the following 2 months, the investigators reported a *"significant improvement"* in depressive symptoms despite the fact that none of the subjects was allowed to keep a pony in his or her bedroom. The average vitamin D level in this group of test subjects went from 16.4 ng/ml (again, pretty low) to 36.4 ng/ml (more like it!). Of course, this makes complete sense. Vitamin D is necessary for proper brain development and function. Vitamin D is also involved in the creation of serotonin, the "feel good" hormone (WebMD, 2008–2011; Patrick and Ames, 2014).

I think it's safe to say that in the future there will be more and more studies pointing to a strong association between low vitamin D levels and childhood depression. It is also reasonable to assume that an association between gestational vitamin D deficiency and depression risk later in life will be uncovered. But I wouldn't wait until more is known about the dangers of vitamin D deficiency before taking action. There are many good reasons to make sure our kids are vitamin D sufficient, both during gestation and after.

Autism

> *Animal data has shown that severe vitamin D deficiency during gestation dysregulates dozens of proteins involved in brain development and leads to rat pups with increased brain size and enlarged ventricles, abnormalities similar to those found in autistic children.* **~Cannell, 2008**
>
> *Vitamin D deficiency, and in particular gestational deficiency, has been implicated in an expanding list of extraskeletal disorders including schizophrenia and autism.* **~Evatt el al., 2009**
>
> *Children born in overcast and rainy counties of Oregon, Washington, and California are twice as likely to be diagnosed with autism as children born in sunnier parts of these states.* **~Patrick and Ames, 2014**

There is definitely more evidence of a relationship between hypovitaminosis D during gestation and autism than there is between hypovitaminosis D and childhood depression. With respect to autism, some say "scanty evidence" (Lucas et al., 2008), others say "tons of evidence" (but in a more sophisticated way). I say, it is so very likely that a relationship between low vitamin D during gestation and autism exists that it is scaring me. Here is why:

- Gestational vitamin D deficiency alters the structure of the fetal brain, in rats and in humans (Féron et al., 2005; Cannell, 2008).

- Autism rates dramatically increased during the time period when sun avoidance was aggressively promoted—heard of sunscreen and its use by women of childbearing age? (Cannell, 2008; Patrick and Ames, 2014).

- Vitamin D is an important neurosteroid, one that promotes factors intimately involved in the development, growth, and survival of neurons within the brain (Féron et al., 2005; Evatt et al., 2009; Patrick and Ames, 2014).

- A drug used to treat epilepsy and known to reduce vitamin D levels, sodium valproate (e.g., Depakote), has been linked to the incidence of autism (Cannell, 2008, Evatt et al., 2009).

- *"It was also noted that children born in winter months, when vitamin D levels are lower, are at increased risk of developing autism."* (Evatt et al., 2009) Similarly, certain regions of the country with lower sunlight availability have a higher rate of autism (Patrick and Ames, 2014)

- Analogous to what has been observed with respect to schizophrenia, there is an increased rate of autism in black immigrants coming from sun-intense regions and moving regions that have comparatively limited sun exposure (Kočovská et al., 2012; Patrick and Ames, 2014).

That's enough. You get the Idea. A relationship between gestational vitamin D deficiency and autism *could* be regarded as strong, perhaps compelling. And let me add: Even if something else, or a combination of things, is found to be *the* cause of autism, do you think gestational vitamin D deficiency is going to help? No, nothing about vitamin D deficiency during fetal development seems to be all that beneficial.

Before we move on, I should probably share this with you: *"Children who have restricted or unusually large fetal growth and those with preterm births have a greater risk for ASD [autism]."* (Lord, 2013) Gestational vitamin D deficiency does all this! It can cause babies to be too small. It can cause babies to be too large. It can cause babies to arrive too early and in trouble.

Psychosis and you name it

> *It is unknown if serum 25OH(D) concentrations in childhood are associated with psychotic experiences.*
>
> *Our findings of an inverse association of 25(OH)D3 with definite psychotic experiences is consistent with the hypothesis that vitamin D may protect against psychosis-related outcomes.* **~Tolppanen et al., 2012b**
>
> *Maternal vitamin D insufficiency during pregnancy is significantly associated with offspring language impairment.* **~Whitehouse et al., 2012**

Again, let's keep this simple. Vitamin D is a hormone involved in the structural development of the brain and is necessary for proper brain function. If vitamin D supplies are low, the brain will face challenges, it could become, and often is, damaged. ***Damaged!*** People can argue all day long as to whether a certain thing, at a certain time, leads to a certain result, and nothing seems to be getting done. There are so many reasons to <u>strenuously</u> promote vitamin D sufficiency, why not add proper brain development to the list and act accordingly. At the very least, vitamin D deficiency during the various stages of brain development is certainly not going to be of any benefit. It is tempting to add attention deficit disorder and intellectual blunting (the story of my life) to the list of problems associated vitamin D deficiency during gestation. Actually, I think someone already has (Morales et al., 2012; Goksugur et al., 2013).

Have I got a book for you!

Several years ago I developed quite an interest in Crohn's disease. So much so that I decided to write a book. Four years of diligence and nearly 500 pages later, it is finally available (almost). The name of the book is ***More to Consider in the Battle against Crohn's***. It will explain, in layman's terms, exactly what this disease is and how it can be treated more effectively. It features the most promising alternative and complementary approaches available for the management of this disease, all meticulously documented. It also contains information useful to individuals suffering from a similar disease called ulcerative colitis. There are surprises in store! This really is a one-of-a-kind book on Crohn's. It only exists because of the careful observations that I have made, the unique experiences that have come my way, and a lot of hard work and dedication. And you know me! I like to share. The book should be available by the end of 2014. I will keep you updated on my website.

Now don't get all excited!

I wish I didn't have to bring this to your attention, but with all the excitement in the air surrounding the legalization of pot, someone needs to issue this warning: Marijuana use will harm you. It will harm your unborn child. Stay away! Say no! Don't make me track you down! ***Do I look like I'm kidding?*** And if I do have to track you down, I'm going to make you read this:

> Research suggests that, at ages three to four years, children of mothers who used marijuana while pregnant have poorer verbal, memory and reasoning ability; poorer motor skills and shorter length of play; and are more likely to be fearful, impulsive, inattentive, hyperactive and delinquent. These difficulties appear to persist to age 10 years, when they may be accompanied by increased depression and anxiety, along with reading and spelling

problems and general underachievement at school. Such deficits may also continue into adolescence and early adulthood, along with an increased risk for initiation of tobacco and marijuana use. (UW Alcohol & Drug Abuse Institute, 2011)

You have no idea of the harm the legalization of pot will do to successive generations, one damaged individual at a time. Well maybe you do now. For more information, go to:

—http://adai.uw.edu/marijuana/factsheets/reproduction.htm
   #sthash.EP1791AX.dpuf

I'm not done. *The sky is falling!*

Evidence is mounting that regular marijuana use increases the chance that a teenager will develop psychosis, a pattern of unusual thoughts or perceptions, such as believing the television is transmitting secret messages. It also increases the risk of developing schizophrenia, a disabling brain disorder that not only causes psychosis, but also problems concentrating and loss of emotional expression.

In one recent study that followed nearly 2,000 teenagers as they became young adults, young people who smoked marijuana at least five times were <u>twice as likely</u> to have developed psychosis over the next 10 years as those who didn't smoke pot. (Harvard Health, 2011, emphasis added)

Chapter 7
Recommendations

Given what we know about the inability to reach the RDAs [recommend daily allowances] for pregnancy from diet, it is important to ensure that all mothers receive at least modest vitamin D supplementation. **~Hyppönen, 2011**

The authors concluded that vitamin D supplementation of 4,000 IU/day for pregnant women is safe and most effective in achieving sufficiency in all women and their neonates. **~Lerchbaum and Obermayer-Pietsch, 2012**

Daily doses of as high as 3,000 IU of vitamin D2 in premature infants, and 4,000 IU in older children, have been used to achieve 25(OH)D levels of 30 to 33 ng/mL without adverse effects. **~Huh and Gordon, 2008**

Vitamin D is important to maternal health, fetal development, and postnatal life. Current prenatal care does not include the monitoring of vitamin D levels, which is an unfortunate oversight because deficiency is easily treated. **~Mulligan et al., 2010**

Although there have been plenty of recommendations scattered throughout this presentation (and placed directly above), I have a few new ones to share with you, and a few that I would like to pay special attention to at this time, focusing primarily upon unique issues that arise during pregnancy. Here they are:

Assume not

Do not assume you are vitamin D sufficient. It is better to assume that you are vitamin D deficient. Most of us are! Pregnancy and nursing increases your need for vitamin D. Make sure it is in adequate supply. And do not assume that your newborn, infant, or child is sufficient in vitamin D. Chances are, he or she is not.

Go ahead

If you are able meet your needs for vitamin D by sensible sun exposure, that's nice! Please, go right ahead. If, on the other hand, you are unable accomplish this consistently and wish to achieve and maintain vitamin D sufficiency by diet, be my guest. But in order to generate the same amount of vitamin D as you would from 20 minutes of sun exposure, you would have to drink 200 glasses of milk (Cannell, 2008). Are you really that thirsty? Think supplementation in relevant amounts.

More is not better

The message of this book is simple: Moms, even kids, need thousands of units of vitamin D per day not hundreds of units per day, according to the experts. And we're are not talkin' mega-dosing of vitamin D here! Yes, compared to 400 units of vitamin D, 4,000 even 6,400 units per day may seem high, but this amount is well within the margin of safety. That being said, it is probably not advisable to supplement higher than this amount on your own. Although up to 10,000 IU per day is considered to be safe (under most circumstances), even by those who are very conservative about vitamin D requirements (Holick, 2011).

Not too much of this!

Do not sunbathe in excess, be realistic. Excessive sun exposure can degrade folic acid (Pérez-López, 2007). You'll need an adequate amount of folic acid to prevent a certain type of birth defect, remember?

Do not—really serious!—take more prenatal vitamin tablets than recommended in a well-meaning attempt to increase your vitamin D intake. You could become vitamin A toxic by doing this, which can even lead to certain birth defects.

Hold the cod-liver oil!—too high in vitamin A. Could be a problem. Besides, cod-liver oil is passé. Have you tasted this stuff!

Shoot for this

The following recommendations seem most reasonable:

A reasonable practice seems to screen pregnant women at risk for hypovitaminosis D to ensure that their serum 25(OH)D level is higher than 30 ng/ml. Risk factors include reduced or inefficient sun exposure (i.e., season, latitude, lifestyle, non-caucasian ethnicity, concealing clothing) or pathological conditions (i.e., malabsorption, liver and kidney disease. (Fanos et al., 2013)

Caution!

Sometimes, the sun can actually harm you, unexpectedly, should certain circumstances exist. Consider this:

UVB irradiation does not appear to suit some individuals who develop headache, nausea and possible vomiting and rise of temperature after exposure. Also people with sensitive skin may react strongly to UV rays, thus are unsuitable for UV treatment.

Certain drugs could make individuals become more susceptible than normal to the effects of UV radiation, examples include gold, sulphonamides, insulin, thyroid extract, and quinine. There UVB should not be used in conjunction with these drugs. (Zhang and Naughton, 2010)

In addition to the above, be aware that a class of diuretics called thiazine diuretic, often used treat high blood pressure, can make one sensitive to higher levels of vitamin D. (Smolders et al., 2008) This could spell trouble. Caution!

Maintain a healthy lifestyle

Obviously, the health of the mother is of paramount importance. How many Red Flags can you spot here?

Multiple health-related behavioral factors have been shown to affect pregnancy outcomes. For example, physical inactivity in mothers is associated with increased risks for obesity and obesity-related chronic conditions such as diabetes mellitus and hypertension, and pregnant women who are obese are at increased risk for miscarriage, pregnancy-induced hypertension and preeclampsia, gestational diabetes, and thromboembolism, and at an increased risk of having children with macrosomia [excessive birth weight], spontaneous intrauterine demises, or delivered by Cesarean section which carries an increased risk for wound infection. Maternal alcohol use and cigarette smoking have been associated with a higher rate of infertility, spontaneous abortion or preterm birth, fetal alcohol syndrome (characterized by growth deficiencies, central nervous system impairment, behavioral disorders, and impaired intellectual devolvement with lifelong implication), and facial dysmorphia [deformity]. Thus, maintaining healthy lifestyles is especially important for women of childbearing age. Previous studies have consistently reported low serum vitamin D concentrations in people with a high BMI [obese] . . . was an independent predictor of vitamin D deficiency and inadequacy among women of childbearing age. Smoking has been associated with a low bone mass and an increased risk for osteoporotic fracture. Brot et al. further reported that middle-aged women who were current smokers had significantly reduced levels of 25(OH)D, $1,25(OH)_2D$ and parathyroid hormone. Our results also showed that smoking was independently associated with vitamin D deficiency in women of childbearing age. However, we found that other behavioral factors such as physical activity and alcohol drinking were not significant determinants of vitamin D status. (Zhao et al., 2012)

Enough of this stuff! How about a few safety rules?

My ten rules of safety

From my extensive review of the research, I have formulated the following ten safety rules for sun exposure and vitamin D supplementation. These apply whether you are pregnant or not. And here they are:

The **first rule** of safety is to not get sunburned, period. ***Period!*** Are we clear? After a reasonable period of sunlight exposure, say 10 minutes to a maximum of 30 minutes (sooner if exposed to intense sunlight), the use of sunscreen is a good call. Aside from protection against sunburning, should you chose the right kind of sunscreen—one that blocks both UVB and UVA rays—excessive UVA rays can promote skin cancer and can give rise to hideous wrinkles (Misra et al., 2008). UVA rays penetrate deeper than UVB rays, and therefore may be more damaging, at least more damaging than previously thought.

Perhaps the **second rule** would be not to take vitamin D in excess. This is why testing is in order. I don't care if you have to pay for it should your insurance company not cover the cost of the 25OHD test. Testing is very important. It will determine how pathetic your vitamin D level really is. Repeated testing will determine if treatment is effective and will help determine your approximate daily need for vitamin D.

The **third rule** is to go slow at first with vitamin D supplementation. I and others believe that prescribing the "rescue" high-dose vitamin D2 protocol (i.e., 50,000 IU/week x 8 to 12 weeks) is not always the best course of action. If this approach is offered to you, a good alternative to suggest would be 10,000 IU/day of D3 for a trial period of several weeks, retest, and then go from there. It may be wise to go slowly at first, with perhaps 1,000 to 2,000 IU/day for a week or two, just to see if you tolerate vitamin D in increased amounts. We have previously discussed a number of medical conditions that warrant caution with vitamin D supplementation (see gray box at the end of *Chapter 5*), so be particularly careful if you fit into this category.

The **fourth rule** is to stop supplementation <u>immediately</u> should you experience any unusual symptom or an increase in disease activity, particularly if you have a chronic illness that you are grappling with. Contact your physician should you believe you are having trouble with vitamin D supplementation.

The **fifth rule** just makes sense. Re-test periodically throughout the year (and particularly after completion of a high-dose treatment regimen). At the very least, get tested during winter to see if you are at a level your physician feels comfortable with. Unless you are faithfully supplementing with vitamin D, and adequately supplementing, a normal vitamin D level in September will not mean that your level will be normal during winter and through the following spring. One test during pregnancy is probably not enough, but one would be better than none.

The **sixth rule** is to take enough vitamin D to do the job. Re-testing is the key here. Some studies suggesting that vitamin D supplementation makes no difference in certain disease states may have been flawed due to the fact that the treated group was simply not given enough vitamin D to do the trick and <u>everybody</u> in the study, including the control group, was actually vitamin D deficient, or vitamin D insufficient at best. Rescue, supplement, then retest. Words to live by.

The **seventh rule** is something my personal physician shared with me. Find a vitamin D supplement of good quality (Hint: not the cheapest) and stick with it. Apparently, not all vitamin D supplements act the same even if the IU are supposed to be the identical. Therefore, if a brand switch occurs, subsequent testing may misinform and make it more difficult to correctly prescribe further dosing. By way of example: If you have a vitamin D level of 52 and you are advised to continue on the 6,000 IU/d, as previously ordered, should you now switch brands, your vitamin D level may drop to, say, 34 and not be at a level the physician is particularly pleased with. (My physician wants my level to be over 50.) I actually had this experience. Taking vitamin D is not rocket science, but it seems reasonable to stick with one brand and one form (D3 vs. D2) so that testing throughout the year will produce more reliable data. Another thing to keep in mind: if you switch from D_3 to D2, a drop in your vitamin D level, too, may occur. And, may I add, D3 has been shown by some to be a better choice than D2 (Armas et al., 2004).

The **eighth rule**: In the summer, and on the summer days you get plenty of sunshine exposure between the hours of 10 AM and 3 PM, you should be able to miss a few days of taking vitamin D supplements. Your excellent, vitamin D-savvy physician will advise you—you have one, right? This brings us to the ninth rule.

The **ninth rule** is one that I just made up, but is certain to find favor with those it the forefront of vitamin D research. This rule states that if your physician is not all that into vitamin D, you must find one who is. Or you have some convincing to do. Hey, why not purchase an extra copy of this book and give it to your physician as a gift? Wrap it up and pretend it is his or her birthday. Put on a funny hat for a prop. (Just a suggestion.)

Safety is undoubtedly a concern with any medication. And, yes, I want you to consider your vitamin D supplement as medication. Clearly, the best approach is to have professional help to make sure you are doing things right. Today, with the availability of 25OHD2 testing, vitamin D supplementation can be tailored to individual need, and it can be done very safely.

Since it seems as though anything that has rules should have at least ten of them to make things sound complete, I guess I'll have to make up one more safety rule.

The **tenth rule** states: If any rule shows up that I did not mention here you can follow it as long as it is a good rule, is simple, and makes perfect sense.

To test or not to test

The only way to determine whether a person is vitamin D . . . sufficient, deficient, or intoxicated is to measure the circulating concentrations of 25(OH)D. **~Holick, 2004a**

As important as the next generation is, of course I am going to recommend testing. And it's a twofer! By testing yourself while you are pregnant, you are also testing your baby. At this point in time, **you** are your baby's <u>only</u> source of vitamin D. If you are deficient, your baby will be deficient. Period! However, due to costs of testing or the belief (disbelief) of some physicians and certain policy makers, it may be tough getting tested. If you cannot afford the test, or for some reason have been convinced that testing is not necessary, ask your OB/GYN if you can follow the 6,400 IU/day recommendation promoted by Hollis and Wagner, a team at the forefront of vitamin D research and maternal/infant need. If there are no contraindications, this would seem to be a reasonable approach and an appropriate request. Remember, there is a wide margin of safety with vitamin D (Vieth et al., 2007). Do you really want to just squeak by with the current recommendation of 600 IU/day of vitamin D along with the little sun exposure that you probably receive? On the other hand, some physicians feel that practically everyone is vitamin D deficient, so why test? Just prescribe. I still think testing is best, particularly for the high-risk individual. (That would be everyone.) Perhaps someone will need "rescued" from a very low vitamin D level. This degree of vitamin D deficiency can <u>only</u> be identified by testing.

There is something about tanning beds

Tanning beds may or may not help you improve your vitamin D status (Holick, 2005). They need to be *UVB-emitting* tanning beds, not the more common *UVA-emitting* tanning beds, in order to generate vitamin D within the skin (Koutkia et al., 2001). The use of a UVB tanning bed has been recommended in cases when there is a malabsorption syndrome in play, one that is preventing the absorption of vitamin D from the gut (Holick, 2004b). Tanning beds work! (see Tangpricha et al., 2004) But be careful! You can "sunburn" in a tanning bed.

And this may come as a surprise

I'm not sure there are many people that know the following, so if you share this with practically anyone, including your physician, this will be sure to impress. Apparently—no, actually—compared to the circulating 25(OH)D3 form, the form of vitamin D made within the skin by a UVB ray, before it can be modified elsewhere, passes more easily into breast milk and right on into the hungry little munchkin (Hollis and Wagner, 2011). So, if it is from sunlight or from a tanning bed, the vitamin D you make, called pre-vitamin D, will be more bioavailable to the nursing infant that the vitamin D obtained from diet or from supplementation. Therefore, a lower vitamin D level in mom may be less of a concern if she is getting at least some of her vitamin D from sun exposure and passing it directly on to her baby one delicious gulp at a time.

Chapter 8
Brand new, and what to do?

Vitamin D deficient mothers will give birth to vitamin D deficient infants. ~**Hyppönen, 2011**

Vitamin D deficiency requires immediate attention and aggressive vitamin D replacement. ~**Holick, 2008**

I am not at all interested in offering medical advice. No, not at all—that's somebody else's job! My job is simply to share with you what this Mommy, Me, and Vitamin D business is all about, and to motivate you to act.

Prevention, of course, is always best, but sometimes this does not occur or it is a little too late. A new little one may find him or herself in a lot of trouble with respect to hypovitaminosis D and will need to be "rescued" right from the start. **A physician will be the one to do this, not you**. The physician, having identified this situation, may want to consider the following:

Muscle function, innate immunity, cellular growth and maturation, insulin secretion, as well as regulation of calcium, phosphorus, and bone metabolism are all affected or controlled by vitamin D. Thus, ensuring that women during pregnancy are vitamin D sufficient and that their newborns either be immediately evaluated for their vitamin D status by measuring 25(OH)D levels in cord blood or given vitamin D prophylactically should be a high priority. Vitamin D deficiency should be immediately treated with at least 1,000 IU of vitamin D2 or vitamin D3/day for the first week of life. Alternately, a single dose of 200,000 IU of vitamin D should suffice for the first few months of life. (Holick, 2006)

Unless you have been supplementing with thousands and not hundreds of units of vitamin D per day during your pregnancy and have obtained only minimal sun exposure, careful screening of your newborn is a must. A blood sample taken from the umbilical cord shortly after birth is all that it takes to determine your baby's vitamin D status. If low, correction is in order. Your baby may look like a healthy newborn, but even this is a Red Flag! He or she may still be severely vitamin D deficient. Wouldn't you want to know? And while you are waiting for the lab results to come back, perhaps this would be an excellent time to discuss the 6,400 IU recommendation of Hollis and Wagner with your physician. You want your breast milk to be up to the task, right? By the way, if your baby is found to be deficient in vitamin D, you will also be degicient. You both may need to be "rescued!"

Perhaps you are very, very late in the game, having paid little if any attention to vitamin D during pregnancy until some time after birth, and you have an ill infant or an ill child on your hands (or six of them— multiple births do happen). By all means, promptly seek medical attention. And please, please, have your baby (or all of them) screened for vitamin D deficiency. Corrective action may be in order. The physician may do well to consider and offer the following advice:

How much sunshine does a baby need? It doesn't take a great deal of sunlight exposure to provide adequate supplies of vitamin D. An infant wearing only a diaper will get enough vitamin D from half an hour per week of sun exposure. A fully clothed infant needs 3 hours. But children with dark skin . . . need more time in the sun. And if parents follow current anticipatory guidance about protecting children from overexposure to the sun and slather on the sunscreen, vitamin D synthesis decreases by more than 95%.

Replenishing vitamin D: Vitamin D deficiency may be remedied by supplementing anywhere along the metabolic pathway. Dihydrotachysterol (DHT, or D1), the substance in the skin that responds to sunlight, is given as 60,000 IU once, then 6000 IU daily until the rickets are clinically and radiologically resolved. Further down-stream, ergocalciferol (D2) may be given as 1000 to 5000 IU daily for 6 to 12 weeks. The dosage is calibrated by age: 1000 IU/d if age <1 month, 3000 IU/d for ages 1 to 12 months, and 5000 IU/d for children older than 12 months. The final form of vitamin D is cholecalciferol (D3). This is typically administered as either 5000 to 10,000 IU daily for 2 to 3 months, or as 600,000 IU in 1 day, divided into 4 to 6 doses. All of these supplements taste bad and children are often resistant to swallowing them. When follow-up and multiple dosing are impractical—because the family finds repeated clinic visits too difficult, or because the child will not comply with the regimen—you can use stosstherapy. This is a bolus of cholecalciferol (D3) or ergocalciferol (D2), 150,000 to 600,000 IU, given as a single dose or divided over several days. For example, you would give 300,000 IU over 1 to 7 days in children 1 to 12 months of age. With this therapy, onset of action is less than a day and maximal effects are seen in 4 weeks. Some preparations contain propylene glycol, which is limited in food additives to <25 mg/kg of body weight because of potential toxicity. (Schmalz et at., 2009)

The above recommendations, offered for consideration <u>by the physician</u>, (sorry for all the big words) would be in keeping with Dr. Holick's call for vitamin D deficiency receiving *"immediate attention and aggressive vitamin D replacement."* (Holick, 2008) Clearly, we simply <u>cannot</u> assume that all is well when it comes to your baby. Remember, the 400 IU of vitamin D in you prenatal is simply not up to the task. Unless you have been obtaining relevant amounts of sun exposure or have been taking thousands of units of vitamin D per day, it is likely that your baby will be deficient, particularly so if you are exclusively breast feeding the new little indoor person.

Out of fear?

Although the medical community has been greatly concerned about vitamin D intoxication, it is one of the rarest reported medical conditions and is usually not observed until >10,000 IU of vitamin D are ingested per day for >5 months. ~**Holick, 2010**

There is a certain reluctance on the part of the physician to treat vitamin D deficiency aggressively. Sometimes little is done. Let's see what Dr. Holick has to say about this. He's the expert on call!

There has been a great fear about causing vitamin D intoxication in neonates. This resulted from the poorly described outbreak of neonatal hypercalcemia [high levels of calcium in the blood] in the 1950s in Great Britain, which led to the enactment of laws in Europe forbidding the fortification of dairy products as well as all other products with vitamin D. In 1997 the Institute of Medicine recommended that the AI [adequate intake] for infants and children of all ages be 200 IU/d. The same recommendation was made for pregnant and lactating women. The safe upper limit for infants ages 0–12 months was 1,000 IU/d and for children older than 1 year of age, 2,000 IU/d. However, it is now obvious based on the historical literature as well as the recent literature that these recommendations are inadequate without sensible sun exposure. It is well documented that neonates and children can tolerate a single dose of 200,000 IU of vitamin D_2 or vitamin D_3 or doses of vitamin D up to 3,000 IU/d without any untoward side effects. Indeed 400–1,000 IU/d to maintain serum 25(OH)D levels between 30–50 ng/ml should be the goal, just as it is in adults. Infants and children have routinely received 400–2,000 IU vitamin D_2 or vitamin D_3/day for the first years of life without any reports of toxicity. Typically, doses of more than 50,000 IU/d of vitamin D_2 were found to cause toxicity.

In Canada, it is recommended that all infants receive 400 IU/d from birth. This recommendation has been successfully implemented and has not resulted in any reported cases of vitamin

D intoxication or hypercalcemia. I believe that the 200 IU of vitamin D that is recommended by the American Academy of Pediatrics is suboptimal. This dose may prevent overt rickets but will not prevent vitamin D deficiency. (Holick, 2006)

Chapter 9
I'm still a little worried about you

Vitamin D should be considered essential for overall health and well-being. Vitamin D deficiency and decreased exposure to solar UVB radiation have been demonstrated to increase the risks of many common cancers, type 1 diabetes, rheumatoid arthritis, and multiple sclerosis, and there are indications that they may be associated with type 2 diabetes and schizophrenia.

Vigilance in maintaining a normal vitamin D status . . . should be a high priority. **~Holick, 2004**

A more recent analysis estimated that **currently between 50,000–63,000 Americans and 19,000–25,000 individuals living in the United Kingdom annually die prematurely from cancer due to vitamin D deficiency**. **~Spina et al., 2006, emphasis added**

Out of fear, I am writing this chapter (actually, out of fear . . . the entire book!).

I am worried about you. So very worried.

I fear that after giving birth you will not have time for yourself— time for hours of youthful sun exposure per week or time for <u>any</u> relevant sun exposure, with a newborn baby and all to take care of. And I worry that your commitment to relevant vitamin D supplementation will wane. It's tough being your favorite author. There is *so much* to worry about. And when I'm not worried about the present, I'm worried about the future.

I worry over your increased risk of cancer should you go through life deficient in vitamin D. Your risk of colon cancer, breast cancer, and ovarian cancer would be <u>substantially</u> increased (Holick, 2005).

I'm deeply worried you may not have the time to read *The Impact of Vitamin D Deficiency*—the best little book that you can buy on, well, the impact of vitamin D deficiency. This, of course, would be most unfortunate. And the following should come as no surprise . . .

When I'm not worried, I am deeply concerned. I am deeply concerned (and worried) about your senior years. Your risk of Alzheimer's, Parkinson's disease, kidney failure, osteoporosis, and hip fracture will be elevated, unless you remain committed to vitamin D sufficiency from now until . . . well, you know.

But before I worry about you in your senior years, I will need to worry about your middle years, the years when your risk of MS, diabetes, Crohn's disease, and rheumatoid arthritis is substantially increased if you are found among those who are, and who remain, vitamin D deficient.

Can you see why I have so much to worry about? I'm even worried that I'm not worried enough! And surprise, surprise . . .

I am so worried that someone will come along and tell you that you need only a few hundred units of vitamin D per day, when, according to the experts, you need thousands of units of vitamin D per day. The real concern here, of course, is that you will believe this notion and lose faith. These are, indeed, perilous times. But I have something else in mind. It's called convincing you of something, and pointing you in the right direction. How am I doing so far?

My goal here is to stop the vicious cycle of vitamin D deficient mothers giving birth to vitamin D deficient babies, babies who grow up vitamin D deficient and become vitamin D deficient mothers with vitamin D deficient aliens inside. What I want is for you to act upon the information contained in this book and become vitamin D sufficient . . . for life! And what I want for your precious little ones is simply that they become vitamin D sufficient, too. Do what it takes. This is all I ask. I am a reasonable man.

The Impact of Vitamin D Deficiency

There, I've gone and done it!—somehow made mention of my other book on vitamin D. Don't know how on earth this slipped in! Now, of course, I'm obliged to tell you more.

Being both concerned and worried, I wrote another nice little book on vitamin D . . . just for you. I wrote this book because I was deeply worried that you were unaware of the destructive force of vitamin D deficiency. This thing kills! And when it is not killing, it is planning on killing. And, while it is not killing or planning on it, it is content with just harming. I am very serious. You have to read this book! Then you will believe. You can purchase *The Impact of Vitamin D Deficiency* on my website or at fine bookstores everywhere (if things go as planned).

—www.impactofvitamind.com

Conclusion

Vitamin D deficiency during pregnancy is the origin for a host of future perils for the child. Some of this damage done by maternal vitamin D deficiency becomes evident after many years. Therefore, prevention of vitamin D deficiency among pregnant women is essential. The current recommended supplementation amount of vitamin D is not sufficient during pregnancy. ~**Kaushal and Magon, 2013, emphasis added**

Vitamin D intake is <u>essential</u> for maternal health and prevention of adverse outcomes. ~**Shin et al., 2010, emphasis added**

In the United states, 25(OH)D$_3$ concentrations are surprisingly low during pregnancy, despite some supplementation with prenatal vitamins. ~**Patrick and Ames, 2014**

Vitamin D is important to maternal health, fetal development, and postnatal life. Current prenatal care does not include the monitoring of vitamin D levels, which is an unfortunate oversight because deficiency is easily treated. ~**Mulligan et al., 2010**

You've seen the evidence. Vitamin D deficiency *is* perilous. Lives are lost, lives are damaged, futures taken away. Deceptively, all appears to be "okay" when supplies are low, and we remain so unaware of the danger. While unaware, we as a society harm ourselves, we harm our mommies, we harm our babies. We harm when we allow vitamin D deficiency to remain commonplace, unidentified, and unresolved. This we could change if we really wanted it to.

Vitamin D is a hormone critical for normal development and function, and for defense. It should be in adequate supply. For the individual, this can only be achieved with generous sun exposure and/or generous vitamin D supplementation. The recommendations of the day do not, will not, <u>cannot</u> stem the tide. These are the recommendations that, if adhered to, will guarantee that we will, over all, remain vitamin D deficient. We the poeple squeak by, and the epidemic continues . . . silently. Mom, you have an important decision or two to make. Will you go forth and do what it takes to make sure that both you and the ones who are depending upon you become and remain vitamin D sufficient? Or will you choose to continue on the path alongside those who are unaware, uninformed, deficient, and who place themselves and their precious little ones in harm's way, unnecessarily? Did I mention someone is counting on you? And did I mention we could sure use a little help?

> The world is currently facing an unrecognized and untreated pandemic of vitamin D deficiency. Sensitizing pediatricians to recognize and treat this pandemic would have great impact on child health in the 21st century. (Rathi and Rathi, 2011)

Need I say more? Probably.

~Acknowledgments~

I wish to thank the following people who helped make this book possible: First and foremost, my dear wife Toni, who encouraged me along the way while I was writing this little book . . . just for you. I extend a special thanks to Gail Leong and Sandy Keno, both medical librarians at Providence Sacred Heart, Spokane, Washington. I also wish to thank my editor and proofreader, Jacquelyn Barnes.

~Appendix~

Recommended websites

There are several websites well worth recommending. Here are my favorites:

- *Vitamin D Council*. **www.vitamindcouncil.org**
  For the latest pregnancy-related information, type "pregnancy" in the website search box.

- *Vitamin D Health.org*. **www.vitamindhealth.org**

- *The Impact of Vitamin D Deficiency* official website
  www.impactofvitamin.com

- *Preventing Birth Defects* official website
  www.preventingbirthdefects.com (still under construction by the author).

~References~

Preface

Holick MF 2003 Vitamin D: A Millennium Perspective. Journal of Cellular Biochemistry 88:296–307

Kaushal M, Magon N 2013 Vitamin D in Pregnancy: A Metabolic Outlook. Indian J Endocrinol Metab; January–February; 17(1):76–82

Introduction

Bener A, Al-Hamaq A OAA, Saleh NM 2013 Association Between Vitamin D Insufficiency and Adverse Pregnancy Outcome: Global Comparisons. International Journal of Women's Health 5:523–531

Cekic M, Cutler SM, VanLandingham JW, Stein DG 2011 Vitamin D Deficiency Reduces the Benefits of Progesterone Treatment after Brain Injury in Aged Rats. Neurobiology of Aging 32:864–874

Grundermann M, von Versen-Höynk F 2011 Vitamin D—Roles in Women's Reproductive Health? Reproductive Biology and Endocrinology 9:146

Kaushal M, Magon N 2013 Vitamin D in Pregnancy: A Metabolic Outlook. Indian J Endocrinol Metab; January–February; 17(1):76–82

Ponsonby A-L, Lucas RM, Lewis S, Halliday J 2010 Vitamin D Status During Pregnancy and Aspects of Offspring Health. Nutrients 2:389–407

Shin JS, Choi MY, Longtine MS, Nelson DM 2010 Vitamin D Effects on Pregnancy and the Placenta. Placenta 31(12):1027–1034

Chapter 1 (Before you know it)

Chaudhuri A 2005 Why We Should Offer Routine Vitamin D Supplementation in Pregnancy and Childhood to Prevent Multiple Sclerosis. Medical Hypothesis 64:608–618

Dror DK, Allen LH 2010 Vitamin D Inadequacy in Pregnancy: Biology, Outcomes, and Interventions. Nutrition Reviews 68(8):465–477

Grayson R, Hewison M 2011 Vitamin D and Human Pregnancy. Food and Maternal Medicine Review 22(1):67–90

Grundermann M, von Versen-Höynk F 2011 Vitamin D—Roles in Women's Reproductive Health? Reproductive Biology and Endocrinology 9:146

Hall JG 2000 Folic Acid: The Opportunity That Still Exists. CMAJ; May 30; 162(11):1571–1572

Hernánadez-Díaz S, Werler MM, Walker AM, Mitchell AA 2001 Neural Tube Defects in Relation to Use of Folic Acid Antagonists during Pregnancy. American Journal of Epidemiology 153(10):961–968

Hulisz D, 2013 Should All Antiepileptic Drugs Be Given with Folic Acid? http://www.medscape.com/view article/814588_print

Kaushal M, Magon N 2013 Vitamin D in Pregnancy: A Metabolic Outlook. Indian J Endocrinol Metab; January–February; 17(1):76–82

Langan RC, Zawistoski KJ 2011 Update on Vitamin D Deficiency. Am Fam Physician 83(12):1425–1430

Lerchbaum E, Obermayer-Pietsch B 2012 Vitamin D and Fertility: A Systematic Review. European Journal of Endocrinology 166:765–778

Lyons RA, Saridogan E, Djahanbakhch O 2006 The Reproductive Significance of Human Fallopian Tube Cilia. Human Reproduction Update 12(4):363–372

Običan SG, Finnell RH, Mills JL, Shaw GM, Scialli AR 2010 Folic Acid in Early Pregnancy: A Public Health Story. FASEB J; November; 24(11):4167–4174

Selhub J, Morris MS, Jacques PF, Rosenberg IH 2009 Folate—Vitamin B-12 Interaction in Relation to Cognitive Impairment, Anemia, and Biochemical Indicators of Vitamin B-12 Deficiency. Am J Clin Nutr 89(suppl):702S–706S

Shin JS, Choi MY, Longtine MS, Nelson DM 2010 Vitamin D Effects on Pregnancy and the Placenta. Placenta 31(12):1027–1034

Silver RM 2007 Fetal Death. Obstetrics & Gynecology; January; 109(1):153–167

Suarez L, Felkner M, Brender JD, Canfield M, Hendricks K 2007 Maternal Exposures of Cigarette Smoke, Alcohol, and Street Drugs and Neural Tube Defect Occurrence in Offspring. Matern Child Health J doi: 10.1007/s10996–007–0251–y

Thompson MD, Cole D EC, Ray JG 2009 Vitamin B-12 and Neural Tube Defects: The Canadian Experience. Am J Clin Nutr 89(suppl):697–701

Van Sande H, Jacquemyn Y, Ajaji M 2013 Vitamin B12 in Pregnancy: Maternal and Fetal/Neonatal Effects—A Review. Open Journal of Obstetrics and Gynecology 3:599–602

WebMD, 2009 Birth Defects Linked to Low Vitamin B12. http://www.webmd.com/baby/news/20090302/birth-defects-linked-to-low-vitamin-b12

WebMD, 2012 Vitamin B12 Deficiency. http://www.webmd.com/food-recipes/guide/vitamin-b12-deficiency-symptoms-causes

Chapter 2 (Everything should be just fine)

Backes CH, Markham K, Moorehead P, Cordero L, Nankervis CA, Giannone PJ 2011 Maternal Preeclampsia and Neonatal Outcomes. Journal of Pregnancy doi: 10.1155/2011/214365

Bener A, Al-Hamaq A OAA, Saleh NM 2013 Association Between Vitamin D Insufficiency and Adverse Pregnancy Outcome: Global Comparisons. International Journal of Women's Health 5:523–531

Ben-Hur H, Gurevich P, Berman V, Tchanyshev R, Gurevich E, Zusman I 2001 The Secretory Immune System As Part of the Placental Barrier in the Second

Trimester of Pregnancy in Humans. *In Vivo*; September–October; 15(5):429–435

Bodnar LM, Catov JM, Simhan HN, Holick MF, Powers RW, Roberts JM 2007a Maternal Vitamin D Deficiency Increases the Risk of Preeclampsia. J Clin Endocrinol Metab 92:3517–3522

Burnam KD 2009 Controversies Surrounding Pregnancy, Maternal Thyroid Status, and Fetal Outcome. Thyroid 19(4):323–326

Burris HH, Rifas-Shinman SL, Kleinman K, Litonjua AA, Huh SY, Rich-Edmonds JW, Camargo Jr CA, Gillman MW 2012 Vitamin D Deficiency in Pregnancy and Gestational Diabetes. Am J Gynecol; September; 207(3):182-e1

Christesen HT, Falkenberg T, Lamont RF, Jørgensen JS 2012 The Impact of Vitamin D on Pregnancy: A Systematic Review. ACTA Obstetrica et Gynecologica 91(2012):1357–1367

Choy MY, Manyonda IT 1998 The Phagocytic Activity of Human First Trimester Extravillous Trophoblast. Human Reproduction 13(10):2941–2949

Cohen MC, Offiah A, Sprigg A, Al-Adnani M 2013 Vitamin D Deficiency and Sudden Unexpected Death in Infancy and Childhood: A Cohort Study. Pediatric and Developmental Pathology 16:292–300

Delange F 2001 Iodine Deficiency as a Cause of Brain Damage. Postgrad Med J 77:217–220

Dover SE, Aroutcheva AA, Faro S, Chikindas ML 2008 Natural Antimicrobials and Their Role in Vaginal Health: A Short Review. Int J Probiotics Prebiotics 3(4):219–230

Dunlop Al, Taylor RN, Tangpricha V, Fortunato S, Menon R 2011 Maternal Vitamin D, Folate, and Polyunsaturated Fatty Acid Status and Bacterial Vaginosis during Pregnancy. Infectious Diseases in Obstetrics and Gynecology doi: 10.1155/2011/216217

Dunn JT, Delange F 2001 Damaged Reproduction: The Most Important Consequence of Iodine Deficiency. The Journal of Clinical Investigation 86(6):2360–2363

Fahey JV, Schaefer TM, Wira CR 2006 Sex Hormone Modulation of Human Uterine Epithelial Cell Immune Responses. Integrative and Comparative Biology 46(6):1082–1087

Fanos M, Vierucci F, Saggese G 2013 Vitamin D in the Prenatal Period: An Update. Journal of Pediatric and Neonatal Individualized Medicine 2(2):e020202

Gillman MW, Rifas-Shiman S, Berkey CS, Field AE, Colditz GA 2003 Maternal Gestational Diabetes, Birth Weight, and Adolescent Obesity. Pediatrics; March; 111(3):e221–e225

Grant WB, Schwalfenberg GK, Gunuis SJ, Whiting SJ 2010 An Estimate of the Economic Burden and Premature Deaths Due To Vitamin D Deficiency in Canada. Mol. Nutr. Food Res 54:1172–1181

Grayson R, Hewison M 2011 Vitamin D and Human Pregnancy. Food and Maternal Medicine Review 22(1):67–90

Grundermann M, von Versen-Höynk F 2011 Vitamin D—Roles in Women's Reproductive Health? Reproductive Biology and Endocrinology 9:146

Huh SY, Gordon CM 2008 Vitamin D Deficiency in Children and Adolescents: Epidemiology, Impact and Treatment. Rev Endocr Metab Disord 9:161–170

Hutton JL, Pharoah POD 2006 Life Expectancy in Severe Cerebral Palsy. Arch Dis Child 91:254–258

Josefson JL, Feinglass J, Rademaker AW, Metzger BE, Zeiss DM, Price HE, Langham CB 2013 Maternal Obesity and Vitamin D Sufficiency Are Associated with Cord Blood Vitamin D Insufficiency. J Clin Endocrinol Metab 98:114–119

Kaushal M, Magon N 2013 Vitamin D in Pregnancy: A Metabolic Outlook. Indian J Endocrinol Metab; January–February; 17(1):76–82

Lain KY, Roberts JM 2002 Contemporary Concepts of the Pathogenesis and Management of Preeclampsia. JAMA; June; 287(4):3183–3186

Liu N, Kaplan AT, Nguyen L, Equils O, Hewison M 2009 Vitamin D Induces Innate Antibacterial Responses in Human Trophoblasts via an Intracrine Pathway. Biology of Reproduction 80:398–406

Liu NQ, Kaplan AT, Lagishetty V, Ouyang YB, Ouyang Y, Simmons CF, Equils O, Hewison M 2011 Vitamin D and the Regulation of Placental Inflammation. The Journal of Immunology 186:5968–5974

March of Dimes 2013 (Last Review) Premature Babies. http:/www.marchofdimes.com/baby/premature-babies.aspx

MD CONSULT 2013 Gabbe: Obstetrics: Normal and Problem Pregnancies, 6th ed. Chapter 35: Hypertension

Mulligan ML, Shaili SK, Riek AE, Bernal-Mizrachi C 2010 Implications of Vitamin D Deficiency in Pregnancy and Lactation. Am J Obstet Gynecol; May; 202(5):429.e1–429.e9

Pérez-López FR 2007 Vitamin D The Secosteroid Hormone and Human Reproduction. Gynecological Endocrinology; January; 23(1):13–24

Ponsonby A-L, Lucas RM, Lewis S, Halliday J 2010 Vitamin D Status During Pregnancy and Aspects of Offspring Health. Nutrients 2:389–407

Post JL, Ernst JZI 2013 Controversies in Vitamin D Recommendations and Its Posible Roles in Nonskeletal Health Issues. J Nutr Food Sci 3(4): doi: 10.4172/2155-9600.1000213

Shand AW, Nassar N, Von Dadelszen P, Innis SM, Green TJ 2010 Maternal Vitamin D Status in Pregnancy and Adverse Pregnancy Outcomes in a Group at High Risk for Preeclampsia. BJOG: An Internal Journal of Obstetrics & Gynaecology 117(13):1593–1598

Shin JS, Choi MY, Longtine MS, Nelson DM 2010 Vitamin D Effects on Pregnancy and the Placenta. Placenta 31(12):1027–1034

Strand Heimstad R, Iversen A-C, Austgulen R, Lydersen S, Andersen GL, Irgens LM, Vik T 2013 Mediators of the Association Between Pre-eclampsia and Ceberal Palsy: Population Based Cohort Study. BMJ: British Medical Journal 347

Thorne-Lyman A, Fawzi WW 2012 Vitamin D During Pregnancy and Maternal, Neonatal and Infant Health Outcomes: A Systematic Review and Meta-Analysis. Paediatric and Perinatal Epidemolology; July; 26(s1): 36–54

Yoon BH, Park C-W, Chaiworapongsa T 2003 Intrauterine Infection and the Development of Cerebral Palsy. BJOG: An International Journal of Obstetrics and Gynaecology; April; 110:124–127

Walsh JM, McGowan CA, Kilbane M, McKenna MJ, McAuliffe FM 2012 the Relationship Between Maternal and Fetal Vitamin D, Insulin Resistance, and Fetal Growth. Reproductive Sciences 20(5):536–541

WebMD 2012 Preeclampsia and Eclampsia. http://www.webmd.com/baby/guide/preeclampsia-eclampsia

WebMD 2013a Understanding Preeclampsia and Eclampsia—the Basics http://www.webmd.com/hypertension-high-blood-pressure/guide/understanding-preeclampsia-eclampsia-basic-information

WebMD,2013b Understanding Preeclampsia and Eclampsia—Symptoms. http://www.webmd.com/baby/understanding-preeclampsia-eclampsia-symptoms

Zhang R, Naughton DP 2010 Vitamin D in Health and Disease: Current Perspectives. Nutrition Journal 9:65

Zuhur SS, Erol RS, Kuzu E, Altuntas Y 2013 The Relationship between Low Maternal Serum 25-Hydroxyvitamin D levels and Gestational Diabetes Mellitus According to the Severity of 25-Hydroxyvitamin D Defeciency. Clinics 68(5):658–664

Chapter 3 (Not up to the task)

Balasubramanian S, Ganesh R 2008 Vitamin D deficiency in Exclusively Breast-fed Infants. Indian J Med Res; March; 127:250–255

Bener A, Al-Hamaq A OAA, Saleh NM 2013 Association Between Vitamin D Insufficiency and Adverse Pregnancy Outcome: Global Comparisons. International Journal of Women's Health 5:523–531

Bodnar LM, Catov JM, Roberts JM, Simhan HN 2007b Prepregnancy Obesity Predicts Poor Vitamin D Status in Mothers and Their Neonates. J. Nutr. 137:2437–2442

Bodnar LM, Simhan HN, Powers RW, Frank MP, Cooperstein E, Roberts JM 2007c High Prevalence of Vitamin D Insufficiency in Black and White Pregnant

Women Residing in the Northern United States and Their Neonates. J. Nutr. 137:447–452

Christesen HT, Falkenberg T, Lamont RF, Jørgensen JS 2012 The Impact of Vitamin D on Pregnancy: A Systematic Review. ACTA Obstetrica et Gynecologica 91(2012):1357–1367

Dawodu A, Wagner CL 2007 Mother-Child Vitamin D Deficiency: An International Perspective. Arch Dis Child 92:737–740

Dominguez-Bello MG, Costello EK, Contreras M, Magris M, Hidalgo G, Fierer N, Knight R 2010 Delivery Mode Shapes the Acquisition and Structure of the Intestinal Microbiota across Multiple Body Habitats in Newborns. Proc Nati Acad Sci USA; June 29; 107(26):11971–11975

Dror DK, Allen LH 2010 Vitamin D Inadequacy in Pregnancy: Biology, Outcomes, and Interventions. Nutrition Reviews 68(8):465–477

Fanos M, Vierucci F, Saggese G 2013 Vitamin D in the Prenatal Period: An Update. Journal of Pediatric and Neonatal Individualized Medicine 2(2):e020202

Grundermann M, von Versen-Höynk F 2011 Vitamin D—Roles in Women's Reproductive Health? Reproductive Biology and Endocrinology 9:146

Hamilton SA, McNeil R, Hollis BW, Davis DJ, Winkler J, Cook C, Werner G, et al 2010 Profound Vitamin D Deficiency in a Diverse Group of Women during Pregnancy Living in a Sun-Rich Environment at Latitude 32°N. Internal Journal of Endocrinology doi: 10.1155/2010/917428

Holick MF 2003 Vitamin D: A Millenium Perspective. Journal of Cellular Biochemistry 88:296–307

Holick MF 2004 Sunlight and Vitamin D for Bone Health and Prevention of Autoimmune Diseases, Cancers, and Cardiovascular Disease. American Journal of Clinical Nutrition; December; 80(6):1678S–1688S

Holick MF 2012 Evidenced-Based D-Bate on Health Benefits of Vitamin D Revisited. Dermatio-Endocrinology; April/May/June; 4(2):183–190

Hollis BW, Wagner CL 2004 Assessment of Dietary Vitamin D Requirements during Pregnancy and Lactation. Am J Clin Nutr 79:717–726

Hyppönen E 2011 Preventing Vitamin D Deficiency in Pregnancy—Importance for the Mother and Child. Annals of Nutrition and Metabolism 59(12):28–31

Kaushal M, Magon N 2013 Vitamin D in Pregnancy: A Metabolic Outlook. Indian J Endocrinol Metab; January–February; 17(1):76–82

Misra M, Pacaud D, Petryk A, Collett-Solberg PF, Kappy M 2008 Vitamin D Deficiency in Children and Its Management: Review of Current Knowledge and Recommendations. Pediatrics 122:398–417

Mulligan ML, Shaili SK, Riek AE, Bernal-Mizrachi C 2010 Implications of Vitamin D Deficiency in Pregnancy and Lactation. Am J Obstet Gynecol; May; 202(5):429.e1–429.e9

Neu J, Rushing J 2011 Cesarean Versus Vaginal Delivery: Long Term Infant Outcomes and the Hygiene Hypothesis. Clin Perinatol; June; 38(2):321–331

Patrick RP, Ames BN 2014 Vitamin D Hormone Regulates Serotonin Synthesis. Part 1: Relevance for Autism. FASEB J 28 [Epub ahead of print]

Rathi N, Rathi A 2011 Vitamin D and Child Health in the 21st Century. Indian Pediatrics 48:619–625

Wagner CL, Taylor SN, Hollis BW 2008 Does Vitamin D Make the World Go "Round"? Breastfeeding Medicine 3(4):239–250

Chapter 4 (To be or not to be)

Bener A, Al-Hamaq A OAA, Saleh NM 2013 Association Between Vitamin D Insufficiency and Adverse Pregnancy Outcome: Global Comparisons. International Journal of Women's Health 5:523–531

Bikle D 2009 Nonclassic Actions of Vitamin D. J Clin Endocrinol Metab 94:26–34

Dawodu A, Wagner CL 2007 Mother-Child Vitamin D Deficiency: An International Perspective. Arch Dis Child 92:737–740

Lerchbaum E, Obermayer-Pietsch B 2012 Vitamin D and Fertility: A Systematic Review. European Journal of Endocrinology 166:765–778

Holick MF 2003 Vitamin D Deficiency: What a Pain It Is. Mayo Clin Proc 78:1457–1459

Holick MF 2005 The Vitamin D Epidemic and Its Health Consequences. J. Nutr. 135:2739S–2748S

Holick MF 2006a High Prevalence of Vitamin D Inadequacy and Implications for Health. Mayoclinicproceedings.com

Holick MF 2006b Resurrection of Vitamin D Deficiency and Rickets. The Journal of Clinical Investigation 116(16):2062–2072

Holick MF 2008 Vitamin D: A D-Lightful Health Perspective. Nutrition Reviews 66(Suppl 2):S182–S194

Holick MF 2010 The Vitamin D Deficiency Pandemic: A Forgotten Hormone Important for Health. Public Health Reviews 32(1):267–283

Holick MF 2012 The D-Lightful Vitamin D for Child Health. Journal of Parenteral and Enteral Nutrition; January; 36(Suppl 1):9S–19S

Hollis BW, Wagner CL 2004 Assessment of Dietary Vitamin D Requirements during Pregnancy and Lactation. Am J Clin Nutr 79:717–726

Huh SY, Gordon CM 2008 Vitamin D Deficiency in Children and Adolescents: Epidemiology, Impact and Treatment. Rev Endocr Metab Disord 9:161–170

Pérez-López FR 2007 Vitamin D The Secosteroid Hormone and Human Reproduction. Gynecological Endocrinology; January; 23(1):13–24

Reichrath J 2007 Vitamin D and the Skin: An Ancient Friend, Revisited. Experimental Dermatology 16:618–625

Wagner CL, Taylor SN, Hollis BW 2008 Does Vitamin D Make the World Go "Round"? Breastfeeding Medicine 3(4):239–250

Chapter 5 (Red flags everywhere!)

Al-Othman A, Al-Musharaf S, Al-Daghri NM, Yakout S, Alkharfy KM, Al-Saleh Y, Al-Attas OS, et al 2012 Tea and Coffee Consumption in Relation to Vitamin D and Calcium Levels in Saudi Adolescents. Nutrition Journal 11:56

Banihossein SZ, Baheiraei A, Shirzad N, Heshmat R, Mohsenifar A 2013 The Effect of Cigarette Smoke Exposure on Vitamin D Level and Biochemical Parameters of Mothers and Neonates. Journal of Diabetes & Metabolic Disorders 12:19

Barnes TC, Bucknall RC 2004 Vitamin D Deficiency in a Patient with Systemic Lupus Erythematosus. Rheumatology 43(3):393–394

Bodnar LM, Catov JM, Roberts JM, Simhan HN 2007b Prepregnancy Obesity Predicts Poor Vitamin D Status in Mothers and Their Neonates. J. Nutr. 137:2437–2442

Carlton-Conway D, Tulloh R, Wood L, Kanabar D 2003 Vitamin D Deficiency and Cardiac Failure In Infancy. Journal of the Royal Society of Medicine; May; 97:238–239

CDC 2013 Medications and Pregnancy. http/www.cdc.gov/pregnancy/meds/

Chesney RW 2008 Rickets or Abuse, or both? Pediatr Radiol doi:10.1007/s00247-008-0993-8

Craig WJ 2009 Health Effects of Vegan Diets. Am J Clin Nutr 89(Suppl):1627S–1633S

Dawodu A, Wagner CL 2007 Mother-Child Vitamin D Deficiency: An International Perspective. Arch Dis Child 92:737–740

Dijkstra SH, van Beek A, Janssen JW, de Vleeschouwer LHM, Huysman WA, van den Akker ELT 2007 High Prevalence of Vitamin D Deficiency in Newborn Infants of High-Risk Mothers. Arch Dis Child 92:750–753

Dror DK, Allen LH 2010 Vitamin D Inadequacy in Pregnancy: Biology, Outcomes, and Interventions. Nutrition Reviews 68(8):465–477

Fakih MG, Trump DL, Johnson CS, Tian L, Muindi J, Sunga AY 2009 Chemotherapy is Linked to Severe Vitamin D Deficiency in Patients with Colorectal Cancer. Int J Colorectal Dis 24:219–224

Fanos M, Vierucci F, Saggese G 2013 Vitamin D in the Prenatal Period: An Update. Journal of Pediatric and Neonatal Individualized Medicine 2(2):e020202

Gracious BL, Finucane TL, Friedman-Campbell M, Messing S, Parkhurst MN 2012 Vitamin D Deficiency and Psychotic Features in Mentally Ill Adolescents: A Cross-Sectional Study. BMC Psychiatry 12:38

Hamilton SA, McNeil R, Hollis BW, Davis DJ, Winkler J, Cook C, Werner G, et al 2010 Profound Vitamin D Deficiency in a Diverse Group of Women during Pregnancy Living in a Sun-Rich Environment at Latitude 32°N. Internal Journal of Endocrinology doi: 10.1155/2010/917428

Hewison M, Adams JS 2009 Vitamin D Insufficiency and Skeletal Development in Utero. Journal of Bone and Mineral Research; January; 25(1):1–3

Holick MF 2004a Sunlight and Vitamin D for Bone Health and Prevention of Autoimmune Diseases, Cancers, and Cardiovascular Disease. American Journal of Clinical Nutrition; December; 80(6):1678S–1688S

Holick MF 2004b Vitamin D: Importance in the Prevention of Cancers, Type 1 Diabetes, Heart Disease, and Osteoporosis. American Journal of Clinical Nutrition; March; 79(3):362–371

Holick MF 2006 Resurrection of Vitamin D Deficiency and Rickets. The Journal of Clinical Investigation 116(16):2062–2072

Holick MF 2007 Vitamin D Deficiency. N Engl J Med; July 19; 357:266–281

Holick MF 2010 The Vitamin D Deficiency Pandemic: A Forgotten Hormone Important for Health. Public Health Reviews 32(1):267–283

Holick MF 2012 The D-Lightful Vitamin D for Child Health. Journal of Parenteral and Enteral Nutrition; January; 36(Suppl 1):9S–19S

Huisman AM, White KP, Algra A, Harth M, Vieth R, Jacobs J, Bulsma J, Bell DA 2001 Vitamin D Levels in Women with Systemic Lupus Erthematosus and Fibromyalgia. J Rheumatol 28:2535–2539

Kaushal M, Magon N 2013 Vitamin D in Pregnancy: A Metabolic Outlook. Indian J Endocrinol Metab; January–February; 17(1):76–82

Keller KA, Barns PD 2008 Rickets vs. Abuse: A National and International Epidemic. Pediatr Radiol doi: 10.1007/s00247–008–1001-z

Lapillonne A 2010 Vitamin D Deficiency during Pregnancy May Impair Maternal and Fetal Outcomes. Medical Hypothesis 74:71–75

Lee K 2012 Sex-Specific Relationships between Alcohol Consumption and Vitamin D Levels: The Korea National Health and Nutrition Survey 2009. Nat Res Pract 6(1):86–90

Misra M, Pacaud D, Petryk A, Collett-Solberg PF, Kappy M 2008 Vitamin D Deficiency in Children and Its Management: Review of Current Knowledge and Recommendations. Pediatrics 122:398–417

Parikh SJ, Edelman M, Uwaifo GI, Freedman RJ, Semega-Janneh M, Reynolds J, Yanovski JA 2004 The Relationship between Obesity and Serum 1,25-Dihydroxy Vitamin D Concentrations in Healthy Adults. The Journal of Endocrinology & Metabolism 89(3):1196–1199

Paterson CR 2009 Vitamin D Deficiency Rickets and Allegations of Non-Accidental Injury. Acta Paediatrica 98(12):2008–2012

Rathi N, Rathi A 2011 Vitamin D and Child Health in the 21st Century. Indian Pediatrics 48:619–625

Schmalz M, Boos K, Schmalz G, Huntington MK 2009 Failure to Thrive. The Journal of Family Practice; October; 58(10):539–544

Schwalfenberg G 2007 Not Enough Vitamin D: Health Consequences for Canadians. Canadian Family Medicine 53:842–854

UCSF Medical Center 2002–2014 Substance Use during Pregnancy. http://www.ucsfhealth.org/education/subsatance_use_during_pregnancy/

*Web*MD 2012 Arthritis: Disease-Modifying Medications
http://www.webmd.com/rheumatoid-arthritis/modifying-
medications?print=true

*Web*MD, 2012 Vitamin B12 Deficiency. http://www.webmd.com/food-
recipes/guide/vitamin-b12-deficiency-symptoms-causes

Wagner CL, Taylor SN, Hollis BW 2008 Does Vitamin D Make the World Go
"Round"? Breastfeeding Medicine 3(4):239–250

Wallis K 2008 Severe Vitamin D Deficiency Presenting as Hypocalcaemic
Seizures in a Black Infant at 45.5 Degrees South: A Case Repost. Cases Journal
1:12 doi: 10.1757/1757–1626–1–12

Whyman JD, Michie C, Chan, Ash S, Carroll R 2010 Muscle Pain and
Hypovitaminosis D in a 10 Year Old Girl: A Case Report. The West London
Medical Journal 2(3):53–75

Wortsman J, Matsuoka LY, Chen TC, Lu Z, Holick MF 2000 Decreased
Bioavailability of Vitamin D in Obesity. Am J Clin Nutr 72:690–693

Zhang R, Naughton DP 2010 Vitamin D in Health and Disease: Current
Perspectives. Nutrition Journal 9:65

Chapter 6 (Spare the children)

American Academy of Allergy Asthma & Immunology 2014 Asthma Statistics
http://www.aaaai.org

American Diabetes Association 2010 Type 1 Diabetes Mortality Rates
Dropping. November 10; www.diabetes.org

**Ananthakrishnan AN, Khalili H, Higuchi LM, Bao Y, Korzenik JR, Giovannucci
EL, Richter JM, et al** 2012 High Predicted Vitamin D Status is Associated with
Reduced Risk of Crohn's Disease. Gastroenterology; March; 142(3):482–489

Arnson Y, Amital H, Shoenfeld Y 2007 Vitamin D and Autoimmunity: New
Aetiological and Therapeutic Considerations. Ann Rheum Dis; June 8; 0:1–6

Battersby AJ, Kampmann B, Burl S 2012 Vitamin D in Early Childhood and the Effects on Immunity to *Mycobacterium Tuberculosis*. Clinical and Developmental Immunology doi: 10.1155/2012/430972

Bener A, Ehlayel MS, Tulic MK, Hamid Q 2012 Vitamin D Deficiency as a Strong Predictor of Asthma. Int Arch Allergy Immunol 157:168–175

Bodnar LM, Catov JM, Simhan HN, Holick MF, Powers RW, Roberts JM 2007a Maternal Vitamin D Deficiency Increases the Risk of Preeclampsia. J Clin Endocrinol Metab 92:3517–3522

Bodnar LM, Simhan HN, Powers RW, Frank MP, Cooperstein E, Roberts JM 2007c High Prevalence of Vitamin D Insufficiency in Black and White Pregnant Women Residing in the Northern United States and Their Neonates. J. Nutr. 137:447–452

Camargo Jr CA, Rifas-Shiman SL, Litonjua AA, Rich-Edwards JW, Weiss ST, Gold DR, Kleinman K, Gillman MW 2007b Maternal Intake of Vitamin D During Pregnancy and Risk of Recurrent Wheeze in Children at 3 y of Age. Am J Clin Nutr 85:788–795

Camargo Jr CA, Ingham T, Wickens K, Thadhani R, Silvers KM, Epton MH, Town I, et al 2011 Cord-Blood 25-Hydroxyvitamin D Levels and Risk of Respiratory Infection, Wheezing, and Asthma. Pediatrics 127:e180–e187

Cannell JJ 2008 Autism and Vitamin D. Medical Hypotheses 70:750–759

Cannell JJ, Vieth R, Umhau JC, Holick MF, Grant WB, Madronich S, Garland CF, Giovannucci E 2011 Epidemic Influenza and Vitamin D. Epidemiol. Infect. 134:1129–1140

Chaudhuri A 2005 Why We Should Offer Routine Vitamin D Supplementation in Pregnancy and Childhood to Prevent Multiple Sclerosis. Medical Hypothesis 64:608–618

Children's Hospital of Wisconsin 2013 Crohn's Disease. http://www.chw.org/display/PPF/DocID/22816/router.asp

Dawodu A, Wagner CL 2007 Mother-Child Vitamin D Deficiency: An International Perspective. Arch Dis Child 92:737–740

Dealberto MJ 2006 Why Are Immigrants at Increased Risk for Psychosis? Vitamin D Insufficiency, Epigenetic Mechanisms, or Both? Medical Hypothesis 68:259–267

Evatt ML, DeLong MR, Grant WB, Cannell JJ, Tangpricha V 2009 Autism Spectrum Disorders following *in utero* Exposure to Antiepileptic Drugs. Neurology; September 22; 73:997

Eyles D, Brown J, Mackay-Sim A, McGrath J, Feron R 2003 Vitamin D and Brain Development. Neuroscience 118:641–653

Eyles DW, Feron F, Cui X, Kesby JP, Harms LH, Ko P, McGrath JJ, Burne THJ 2009 Developmental Vitamin D Deficiency Causes Abnormal Brain Development. Psychoneuroendocrinology 34S:S247–S257

Féron F, Burne THJ, Brown J, Smith E, McGrath JJ, Mackay-Sim A, Eyles DW 2005 Developmental Vitamin D_3 Deficiency Alters the Adult Rat Brain. Brain Research Bulletin 65:141–148

Goksugur SB, Tufan AE, Semiz M, Gunes C, Bekdas M, Tosun M, Demircioglu F 2013 Vitamin D Status in Children with Attention Deficit Hyperactivity Disorder. Pediatrics International doi: 10.1111/ped.12286

Gombart AF 2009 The Vitamin D-Antimicrobial Peptide Pathway and Its Role in Protection against Infection. Future Microbiol; November; 4:1151–1165

Harris SS 2005 Vitamin D in Type 1 Diabetes Prevention. J. Nutr. 135:323–325

Harvard Health 2011 Teens Who Smoke Pot at Risk for Later Schizophrenia Psychosis. Harvard Health Blog; March 7, 2011, 11:03 am

Hviid A, Svanström H, Frisch M 2011 Antibiotic Use and Inflammatory Bowel Disease. Gut 60:49–50

Holick MF 2002 Vitamin D: The Unappreciated D-Lightful Hormone that is Important for Skeletal and Cellular Health. Current Opinion in Endocrinology & Diabetes 9:87–98

Holick MF 2005 The Vitamin D Epidemic and Its Health Consequences. J. Nutr. 135:2739S–2748S

Holick MF 2006 Resurrection of Vitamin D Deficiency and Rickets. The Journal of Clinical Investigation 116(16):2062–2072

Holick MF 2007 Vitamin D Deficiency. N Engl J Med; July 19; 357:266–281

Holick MF 2012 The D-Lightful Vitamin D for Child Health. Journal of Parenteral and Enteral Nutrition; January; 36(Suppl 1):9S–19S

Hollis BW, Johnson D, Hulsey TC, Ebeling M, Wagner CL 2011 Vitamin D Supplementation During Pregnancy: Double Blind, Randomized Clinical Trial of Safety and Effectiveness. Journal of Bone and Mineral Research; October; 26(10):2341–2357

Högberg C, Gustarsson SA, Hällström T, Gustafsson T, Klawitter B, Peterson M 2012 Depressed Adolescents in a Case-Series Were Low In Vitamin D and Depression Was Ameliorated by Vitamin D Supplementation. Acta Paediatrica 101:779–783

Islam T, Gauderman WJ, Cozen W, Mack TM 2007 Childhood Sun Exposure Influences Risk of Multiple Sclerosis in Monozygotic Twins. Neurology 69:381–388

Kaushal M, Magon N 2013 Vitamin D in Pregnancy: A Metabolic Outlook. Indian J Endocrinol Metab; January–February; 17(1):76–82

Kelsall BL 2008 Innate and Adaptive Mechanisms to Control Pathological Intestinal Inflammation. J Pathol 214:242–259

Kiraly ST, Kiraly MA, Hawe RD, Makhani N 2006 Vitamin D as a Neuroactive Substance: Review. The Scientific World Journal 6:125–139

Knip M, Veijola R, Virtanen SM, Hyöty H, Vaarala O, Åkerblom HK 2005 Environmental Triggers and Determinates of Type 1 Diabetes. Diabetes 54(Suppl 2):S125–S136

Kočovská E, Fernell E, Billstedt E, Minnis H, Gillberg C 2012 Vitamin D and Autism: Clinical Review. Research in Developmental Disabilities 33:1541–1550

Laaksi I, Ruohola J-P, Mattila V, Auvinen A, Ylikomi T, Pihlajamäki H 2010 Vitamin D Supplementation for the Prevention of Acute Respiratory Tract Infection: A Randomized, Double-Blinded Trial among Young Finnish Men. The Journal of Infectious Diseases 202(5):809–814

Lange NE, Litonjua A, Hawrylowicz CM, Weiss S 2009 Vitamin D, the Immune System and Asthma. Expert Rev Clin Immunol; November; 5(6):693–702

Levenson CW, Figuerôa SM 2008 Gestational Vitamin D Deficiency: Long-Term Effects on the Brain. Nutritional Reviews 66(12):726–729

Litonjua AA 2009 Childhood Asthma May be a Consequence of Vitamin D Deficiency. Curr Opin Allergy Immunol; June; 9(3):202–207

Liu N, Kaplan AT, Nguyen L, Equils O, Hewison M 2009 Vitamin D Induces Innate Antibacterial Responses in Human Trophoblasts via an Intracrine Pathway. Biology of Reproduction 80:398–406

Lord C 2013 Fetal and Sociocultural Environments and Autism. Am J Psychiatry; April; 170(4):355–358

Lucas RM, Ponsonby A-L, Pasco JA, Morley R 2008 Future Health Implications of Prenatal and Early-Life Vitamin D. National Reviews 66(12):710–720

Markham JA, Koenig JI 2011 Prenatal Stress: Role in Psychotic and Depressive Diseases. Psychopharmacology 214(1):89–106

Mathieu C, Badenhoop K 2005 Vitamin D and Type 1 Diabetes Mellitus: State of the Art. Trends in Endocrinology and Metabolism; August; 16(6):261–265

McCann JC, Ames BN 2008 Is There Convincing Biological or Behavioral Evidence Linking Vitamin D Deficiency to Brain Dysfunction? FASEB J.22:982–1001

McGrath J 1999 Hypothesis: Is Low Prenatal Vitamin D a Risk Factor for Schizophrenia. Schizophrenia Research 40:173–177

McGrath J, Saari K, Hakko H, Jokelainen J, Jones P, Järvelin M-R, Chant D, Isohanni M 2004 Vitamin D Supplementation During the First Year of Life and Risk of Schizophrenia: A Finnish Birth Cohort Study. Schizophrenia Research 67:3237–3245

Medscape Medical News 2012 Vitamin D May Decrease Risk for Crohn's Disease. http://www.medscape.com/viewarticle/759599-print

Misra M, Pacaud D, Petryk A, Collett-Solberg PF, Kappy M 2008 Vitamin D Deficiency in Children and Its Management: Review of Current Knowledge and Recommendations. Pediatrics 122:398–417

Morales E, Guxens M, Llop S, Rodriguez-Bernal CL, Tardón A, Riaño I, Ibarluzea J, et al 2012 Circulating 25-Hydroxyvitamin D_3 in Pregnancy and Infant Neuropsychological Development. Pediatrics; October; 130(4):e913–e920

Munger KL, Levin LI, Hollis BW, Howard NS, Ascherio A 2006 Serum 25-Hydroxyvitamin D Levels and Risk of Multiple Sclerosis. JAMA; December 20; 296(23):2832–2838

MultipleSclerosis.net 2012–2014 MS Statistics. http://Multiplesclerosis.net/what-is-ms-statistics/

Nerich V, Jantchou P, Boutron-Ruault M-C, Weill A, Vanbockstael V, Auleley G-R, Balaire C, et al 2011 Low Exposure to Sunlight Is a Risk Factor for Crohn's Disease. Aliment Pharmacol Ther 33:940–945

Patrick RP, Ames BN 2014 Vitamin D Hormone Regulates Serotonin Synthesis. Part 1: Relevance for Autism. FASEB J 28 [Epub ahead of print]

Rathi N, Rathi A 2011 Vitamin D and Child Health in the 21st Century. Indian Pediatrics 48:619–625

Shand AW, Nassar N, Von Dadelszen P, Innis SM, Green TJ 2010 Maternal Vitamin D Status in Pregnancy and Adverse Pregnancy Outcomes in a Group at High Risk for Preeclampsia. BJOG: An Internal Journal of Obstetrics & Gynaecology 117(13):1593–1598

Shaw SY, Blanchard JF, Bernstein CN 2010 Association Between the Use of Antibiotics in the First Year of Life and Pediatric Inflammatory Bowel Disease. The American Journal of Gastroenterology 105(12):2687–2692

Staples J, Ponsonby A-L, Lim L 2010 Low Maternal Exposure to Ultraviolet Radiation in Pregnancy, Month of Birth, and Risk of Multiple Sclerosis in Offspring: Longitudinal Analysis. BMJ doi: 10.1136/bmj.c1640

Tariq MM, Streeten EA, Smith HA, Sleemi A, Khabazghazvini B, Vaswani D, Postolache TT 2011 Vitamin D: A Potential Role in Reducing Suicide Risk. Int J Adolesc Med Health 23(3):157–165

Tolppanen A-M, Sayers A, Fraser WD, Lewis G, Zammit S, Lawlor DA 2012a The Association of Serum 25-hydroxyvitamin D_3 and D_2 with Depressive Symptoms in Childhood—A Prospective Cohort Study. Journal of Child Psychology and Psychiatry 53(7):757–766

Tolppanen A-M, Sayers A, Fraser WD, Lewis G, Zammit S, McGrath J, Lawlor DA 2012b Serum 25-hydroxyvitamin D_3 and D_2 and Non-Clinical Psychotic Experiences in Childhood. PLoS ONE; July; 7(7):e41575

UW Alcohol & Drug Abuse Institute 2011 (last update) Marijuana and Reproduction/Pregnancy.
http://adai.washington.edu/marijuana/factsheets/reproduction.pdf

Vieth R, Bischoff-Ferrari H, Boucher BJ, Dawson-Hughes B, Garland CR, Heaney RP, Holick MF, et al 2007 The Urgent Need to Recommend an Intake of Vitamin D that is Effective. Am J Clin Nutr 85:649–650

Walker VP, Modlin RL 2009 The Vitamin D Connection to Pediatric Infections and Immune Function. Pediatr Res; May; 65(5 Pt 2): 106R–113R

*Web*MD 2008–2011 Serotonin: 9 Questions and Answers
http://www.webmd.com/depression/features/serotonin

*Web*MD 2012 Depression in Children.
http://www.webmd.com/depression/guide/depression-children

*Web*MD 2013 MS (Multiple Sclerosis) in Children.
http://www.webmd.com/multiple-sclerosis/ms-in-children

Whitehouse AJO, Holt BJ, Serralha M, Holt PG, Kusel MMH, Hart PH 2012
Maternal Serum Vitamin D Levels During Pregnancy and Offspring
Neurocognitive Development. Pediatrics 129:485—483

Yamamoto-Furusho JK, Korzenik JR 2006 Crohn's Disease: Innate
Immunodeficiency? World J Gastroenterol; November 14; 12(42):6751–6755

Zhao G, Ford ES, Tsai J, Li C, Croft JB 2012 Factors Associated with Vitamin D
Deficiency and Inadequacy among Women of Childbearing Age in the United
States. ISRN Obstetrics and Gynecology Article ID 691486 doi:
10.5402/2012/691486

Zittermann A, Schleithoff SS, Tenderich G, Berthold HK, Körfer R, Stehle P
2003 Low Vitamin D Status: A Contributing Factor in the Pathogenesis of
Congestive Heart Failure? J Am Coll Cardiol 41:105–112

Chapter 7 (Recommendations)

Cannell JJ 2008 Autism and Vitamin D. Medical Hypotheses 70:750–759

Fanos M, Vierucci F, Saggese G 2013 Vitamin D in the Prenatal Period: An
Update. Journal of Pediatric and Neonatal Individualized Medicine
2(2):e020202

Holick MF 2004a Sunlight and Vitamin D for Bone Health and Prevention of
Autoimmune Diseases, Cancers, and Cardiovascular Disease. American Journal
of Clinical Nutrition; December; 80(6):1678S–1688S

Holick MF 2004b Vitamin D: Importance in the Prevention of Cancers, Type 1
Diabetes, Heart Disease, and Osteoporosis. American Journal of Clinical
Nutrition; March; 79(3):362–371

Holick MF 2005 The Vitamin D Epidemic and Its Health Consequences. J. Nutr.
135:2739S–2748S

Holick MF 2011 The D-Batable Institute of Medicine Report: A D-Lightful Perspective. Endocrine Practice; January/February; 17(1):143–149

Hollis BW, Wagner CL 2011 The Vitamin D Requirements during Human Lactation: The Facts and IOM's "Utter" Failure. Public Health Nutrition 14(4):748–749

Hollis BW, Johnson D, Hulsey TC, Ebeling M, Wagner CL 2011 Vitamin D Supplementation During Pregnancy: Double Blind, Randomized Clinical Trial of Safety and Effectiveness. Journal of Bone and Mineral Research; October; 26(10):2341–2357

Huh SY, Gordon CM 2008 Vitamin D Deficiency in Children and Adolescents: Epidemiology, Impact and Treatment. Rev Endocr Metab Disord 9:161–170

Hyppönen E 2011 Preventing Vitamin D Deficiency in Pregnancy—Importance for the Mother and Child. Annals of Nutrition and Metabolism 59(12):28–31

Koutkia P, Lu Z, Chen TC, Holick MF 2001 Treatment of Vitamin D Deficiency Due to Crohn's Disease with Tanning Bed Ultraviolet B Radiation. Gastroenterology 122:1485–1488

Lerchbaum E, Obermayer-Pietsch B 2012 Vitamin D and Fertility: A Systematic Review. European Journal of Endocrinology 166:765–778

Misra M, Pacaud D, Petryk A, Collett-Solberg PF, Kappy M 2008 Vitamin D Deficiency in Children and Its Management: Review of Current Knowledge and Recommendations. Pediatrics 122:398–417

Mulligan ML, Shaili SK, Riek AE, Bernal-Mizrachi C 2010 Implications of Vitamin D Deficiency in Pregnancy and Lactation. Am J Obstet Gynecol; May; 202(5):429.e1–429.e9

Pérez-López FR 2007 Vitamin D The Secosteroid Hormone and Human Reproduction. Gynecological Endocrinology; January; 23(1):13–24

Smolders J, Damoiseaux J, Menheere P, Hupperts R 2008 Vitamin D as an Immune Modulator in Multiple Sclerosis, A Review. Journal of Neuroimmunology 194:7–17

Tangpricha V, Turner A, Spina C, Decastro S, Chen TC, Holick MF 2004 Tanning Is Associated with Optimal Vitamin D Status (Serum 25-hydroyvitamin D Concentration) and Higher Bone Mineral Density. Am J Clin Nutr 80:1645–1649

Vieth R, Bischoff-Ferrari H, Boucher BJ, Dawson-Hughes B, Garland CR, Heaney RP, Holick MF, et al 2007 The Urgent Need to Recommend an Intake of Vitamin D that is Effective. Am J Clin Nutr 85:649–650

Zhang R, Naughton DP 2010 Vitamin D in Health and Disease: Current Perspectives. Nutrition Journal 9:65

Zhao G, Ford ES, Tsai J, Li C, Croft JB 2012 Factors Associated with Vitamin D Deficiency and Inadequacy among Women of Childbearing Age in the United States. ISRN Obstetrics and Gynecology Article ID 691486 doi: 10.5402/2012/691486

Chapter 8 (New, and what to do)

Holick MF 2006 Resurrection of Vitamin D Deficiency and Rickets. The Journal of Clinical Investigation 116(16):2062–2072

Holick MF 2008 Vitamin D: A D-Lightful Health Perspective. Nutrition Reviews 66(Suppl 2):S182–S194

Holick MF 2010 The D-lemma: To Screen or Not to Screen for 25-Hydroxyvitamin D Concentrations. Clinical Chemistry 56(5):729–731

Hyppönen E 2011 Preventing Vitamin D Deficiency in Pregnancy—Importance for the Mother and Child. Annals of Nutrition and Metabolism 59(12):28–31

Schmalz M, Boos K, Schmalz G, Huntington MK 2009 Failure to Thrive. The Journal of Family Practice; October; 58(10):539–544

Chapter 9 (I'm still a little worried about you)

Holick MF 2004 Sunlight and Vitamin D for Bone Health and Prevention of Autoimmune Diseases, Cancers, and Cardiovascular Disease. American Journal of Clinical Nutrition; December; 80(6):1678S–1688S

Holick MF 2005 The Vitamin D Epidemic and Its Health Consequences. J. Nutr. 135:2739S–2748S

Spina CS, Tangpricha V, Uskokovic M, Adorinic L, Maehr H, Holick MF 2006 Vitamin D and Cancer. Anticancer Research 26:2515–2524

Conclusion

Mulligan ML, Shaili SK, Riek AE, Bernal-Mizrachi C 2010 Implications of Vitamin D Deficiency in Pregnancy and Lactation. Am J Obstet Gynecol; May; 202(5):429.e1–429.e9

Rathi N, Rathi A 2011 Vitamin D and Child Health in the 21st Century. Indian Pediatrics 48:619–625

Shin JS, Choi MY, Longtine MS, Nelson DM 2010 Vitamin D Effects on Pregnancy and the Placenta. Placenta 31(12):1027–1034